FARM ANIMALS DISEASES, RECENT OMIC TRENDS AND NEW STRATEGIES OF TREATMENT

Edited by **Rosa Estela Quiroz-Castañeda**

Farm Animals Diseases, Recent Omic Trends and New Strategies of Treatment
http://dx.doi.org/10.5772/63390
Edited by Rosa Estela Quiroz-Castañeda

Contributors

Rosa Estela Quiroz Castañeda, Fernando Martinez, Bernardo Sachman-Ruiz, Estefan Miranda Miranda, Hugo Aguilar-Diaz, Ramón Alberto Batista-García, Juan Mosqueda, Sergio D. Rodríguez- Camarillo, Mayra E. Cobaxin-Cárdenas

Published by InTech
Janeza Trdine 9, 51000 Rijeka, Croatia

Publishing Process Manager Romina Rovan
Technical Editor SPi Global
Cover InTech Design team

First published March, 2018
Printed in Croatia
Legal deposit, Croatia: National and University Library in Zagreb

Additional hard copies can be obtained from orders@intechopen.com

Farm Animals Diseases, Recent Omic Trends and New Strategies of Treatment, Edited by Rosa Estela Quiroz-Castañeda
p. cm.
Print ISBN 978-953-51-3911-9
Online ISBN 978-953-51-3912-6

For EU product safety concerns:
IN TECH d.o.o., Prolaz Marije Krucifikse Kozulić 3, 51000 Rijeka, Croatia,
info@intechopen.com or visit our website at intechopen.com.

Meet the editor

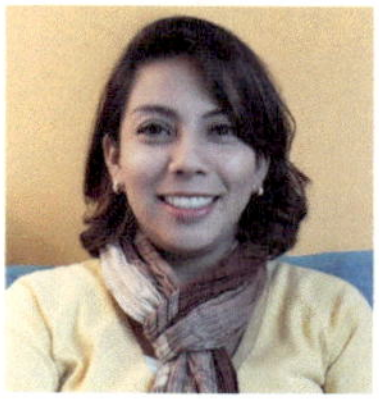

Dr. Rosa Estela Quiroz-Castañeda graduated from the Sciences Faculty of Autonomous University of Morelos in 2003. She received her MS degree in Biochemical Sciences from the National Autonomous University of México (UNAM) in 2005 and PhD degree from the same University in 2011. Currently, she is a full researcher at the National Center for Disciplinary Research in Veterinary Parasitology (CENID-PAVET)-INIFAP in Morelos, México. She has experience in microbial biotechnology, molecular biology, and recently, diagnosis and characterization of pathogens and bacterial genomics, especially those of pathogens of veterinary interest such as *Anaplasma marginale* and *Candidatus Mycoplasma haemobos*. Her research is focused on livestock genomics as a useful tool to identify potential molecules of Rickettsial pathogens and hemoplasmas that have potential as immunogens.

Contents

Preface

Animal health is constantly threatened by pathogens that humans must control to avoid significant losses. The study of these pathogens using omic approaches has revealed valuable information that may contribute to control and prevent diseases. Subsequently, new strategies of treatment might be used instead of those based on chemicals.

This book presents the recent advances in the omic field focused on pathogens of veterinary interest, including *Anaplasma marginale*, *Babesia* spp., *Eimeria* spp., and rickettsiae, among others. The aim of this work is to present a general view of those diseases affecting the farm animals and how omic sciences can contribute to veterinary interest.

The first chapter focuses on the use of bioinformatic tools for the molecular identification of pathogens and their virulence factors. The results of the pathogenomic analysis are the basis for designing new strategies of treatment mediated by vaccines.

The second chapter contains a profound analysis of ticks' immune response, which might lead to a better understanding of how ticks cope with the presence of pathogens.

Chapters three and four contain information about genomic approaches and vaccinology as alternatives to vaccines developed for bovine anaplasmosis and babesiosis. The genomic information of these pathogens and vaccinology is presented as a powerful combination applied to tick-borne diseases.

Rickettsioses are considered as emergent diseases. In the last year, significant information generated by genomic sequencing has been reported. Chapter five presents the genomic analyses of rickettsiae and how this information can drive the development of new prevention strategies, especially due to rickettsiae, which bacteria can be transmitted by ticks from domestic animals to humans.

Other pathogens with veterinary interest are members of phylum Apicomplexa. In chapter six, the genomic approaches to these pathogens are revised.

The use of natural compounds is widely reported to control farm diseases, including avian coccidiosis. Chapters seven and eight present the efforts made to obtain natural products that can be used to control pathogens, such as essential oils and herbal extracts. Avian coccidiosis is one of the most important diseases in poultry, which effects can be treated with natural compounds.

Since pathogens can be transmitted directly to humans, the interest for zoonoses has grown. In Chapter nine we present a special topic about the zoonotic trematodiasis.

Finally, in chapter ten, authors present how metagenomic analyses can characterize the microbiomes and viromes uncultured under laboratory conditions.

In summary, this book aims to emphasize how these omic analyses have led researchers to know many mechanisms that pathogens use to invade and colonize the host cell of farm animals. With this information, new diagnosis, prevention, and treatment strategies could be developed in the future.

Rosa Estela Quiroz-Castañeda, PhD
Anaplasmosis Unit
National Center for Disciplinary Research in Veterinary Parasitology
(CENID-PAVET)-INIFAP
Jiutepec, Morelos, México

Chapter 1

Pathogenomics and Molecular Advances in Pathogen Identification

Rosa Estela Quiroz-Castañeda

Additional information is available at the end of the chapter

http://dx.doi.org/10.5772/intechopen.73695

Abstract

Today exists a spread spectrum of tools to be used in pathogen identification. Traditional staining and microscopic methods as well as modern molecular methods are presented in this chapter. Pathogen identification is only the beginning to obtain information related to pathogenicity of the microorganism in the near future. Once the pathogen is identified, genome-sequencing methods will provide a significant amount of information that can be elucidated only through bioinformatics methods. In this point, pathogenomics is a powerful tool to identify potential virulence factors, pathogenicity islands, and many other genes that could be used as therapeutic targets or in vaccine development. In this chapter, we present an update of the molecular advances used to identify pathogens and to obtain information of their diversity. We also review the most recent studies on pathogenomics with a special attention on pathogens of veterinary importance.

Keywords: pathogenomics, pathogen identification, phylogeny, genome sequencing, infectious diseases

1. Introduction

Infectious diseases not only represent one of the biggest threats to public health but also to animal health and welfare. A significant number of pathogenic microorganisms can be transmitted by vectors; among these, vector-borne pathogens are considered important since they can spread easily pathogens to previously pathogen-free livestock areas [1].

Nowadays, we can identify cultured or non-cultured organisms with molecular techniques and even reconstruct a phylogeny to propose a new species or reclassify reported microorganisms.

Molecular identification methods offer some advantages as being more sensitive and quicker than traditional culture methods at relatively low cost. Many microorganisms are difficult to culture or noncultured which difficult their study *in vitro,* this is overcome by using genome sequencing as an alternative [2].

Currently, the high-throughput next generation sequencing (HT-NGS) technologies have provided a huge amount of information in genomics researches [3]. Genome sequencing and new omics studies, such as pathogenomics, reveal a new landscape of study of microorganisms and reveal unexpected aspects of pathogen biology. These studies have brought a re-evaluation of definitions of pathogens and virulence factors [4].

In order to understand the complex interaction established between host-pathogen, several genomes of farm animals are sequenced (http://www.ensembl.org/info/about/species.html): cat (*Felis catus*), chicken (*Gallus gallus*), cow (*Bos taurus*), dog (*Canis lupus familiaris*), horse (*Equus caballus*), pig (*Sus scrofa*), sheep (*Ovis aries*), turkey (*Meleagris gallopavo*), and duck (*Anas platyrhynchos*).

However, a scarce number of reports are focused on studying pathogenomics of microorganisms affecting farm animals, a field with a high potential to provide new insights to understand pathogen-host interaction from an omic point of view. The new omics techniques applied in veterinary studies provide a new landscape for research in order to elucidate the mechanisms that pathogens employ to develop infection, and then try to develop new mechanisms of control and treatment.

2. Pathogenomics

Molecular identification methods afford for culturable and non-culturable pathogens' identification; however, the entire genome information remains unknown. High-throughput sequencing technologies have opened the possibility to get access to valuable information contained in the genome [5].

Pathogenomics is a discipline that seeks to mark out virulence factors and their contributions to overall pathogenesis by comparing gene repertoires of pathogenic and non-pathogenic strains/species [4].

Today, sequencing and comparing genomes of several strains of a single pathogen is a relatively short time process [6]. One of the crucial genomic analyses is driven to understand microorganisms' pathogenicity and virulence through intensive and refined bioinformatics tools.

Over the years, the genomics information has changed the concept of a static microbial genome and has demonstrated that bacterial genomes are in a dynamic process. The bacterial genome dynamics is driven basically by three forces: gene gain, gene loss, and gene change, and these three forces comprise of several factors affecting bacterial genome dynamics, such as gene duplication, single-nucleotide polymorphism (SNPs), horizontal gene transfer (HGT), recombination and rearrangements, among others (**Figure 1**) [4, 6].

http://dx.doi.org/10.5772/intechopen.73695

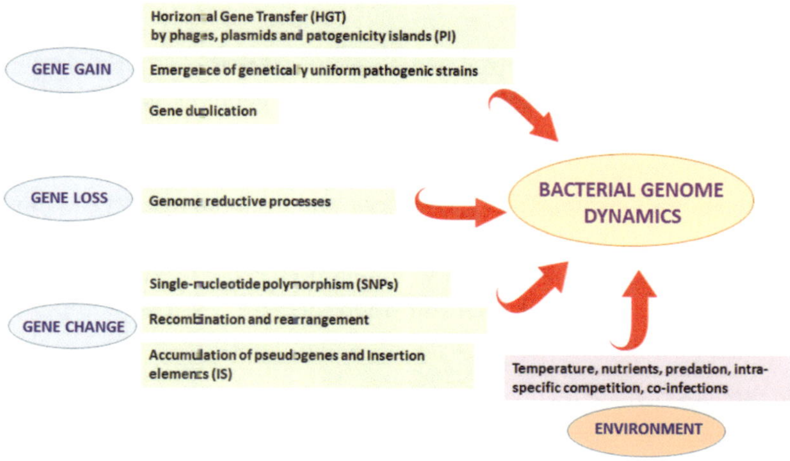

Figure 1. Gene gain, gene loss, gene change, and the environment are the main factors influencing on bacterial genome dynamics.

The smallest variation in bacterial genomes is the SNPs, which have been detected more recently by whole-genome sequencing. Sondgeroth et al. [7] used SNPs of five genes to monitor potential changes in the *B. bovis* population composition before and after passage through the tick vector. A substantial polymorphism among *F. hepatica* isolates was observed by Cwiklinski et al. [8], and they found that 48% of genes exhibited at least one non-synonymous SNP, and these genes were associated with biological processes as axonogenesis and chemotaxis.

2.1. Pathogenomics studies

In order to address what makes bacteria pathogenic is important to know the functional differences between pathogenic and non-pathogenic strains or species. Nowadays, the number of sequenced genomes increases constantly and this has made feasible comparative analyses between pathogenic and non-pathogenic bacterial genomes.

A significant variation in size and content of genomes between different genera and species, and even in strains of the same species has been reported [6].

Pathogenicity is an ability of an organism to cause disease and microorganisms possess several factors that enable them to increase their virulence or degree of pathogenicity.

Toxicity and invasiveness are the two properties of pathogens to cause disease; the first one refers to degree to which a substance causes harm and the latter is the ability to penetrate into the host and then spread [9]. Host and pathogens have co-evolved over millions of years and in this relationship, pathogens have modified their virulence to adapt to the host immune system.

Due to gain or loss of genes pathogens adapting to the changing environments, in this sense, genomic studies are indispensable to identify differences between genomes to provide invaluable insights into virulence and pathogenesis [10].

2.1.1. Mobile genetic elements (MGE)

The term MGE encompasses specialized genetic elements that play a role in genomic instability including plasmids, bacteriophages, transposons, genomic islands (GI), inteins, introns, retroelements and integrons, and many other specialized genetic elements such as insertion sequence elements (IS), miniature inverted-repeat transposable elements [MITEs], repetitive extragenic palindromic [REP] sequences, and bacterial interspread mosaic element [BIMEs] [11]. Among bacterial strains exist a particular interest due to the presence of virulence factors that may be introduced to a new host genome. As MGE are involved in genomic rearrangements and virulence acquisition they are considered important elements in bacterial genome evolution [12].

MGE encode proteins that are involved in cell surface structures (capsular polysaccharides, O-antigen, S-layer, flagella, pilli, and porins) and toxins [10]. Type II and type III toxin-antitoxin systems (TASs) belong to the class of bacterial MGEs that are spread by horizontal gene transfer and they appear to behave like selfish elements contributing to the stable maintenance and dissemination of plasmids and genomic islands in bacterial populations [13]. Here, we will focus on explaining some of the features of IS, GIs, and PAIs.

2.1.1.1. Insertion sequences (IS)

IS elements represents an important component of most bacterial genomes; they usually have a size of ranging from 0.7 to 3.5 kB, including a transposase gene encoding the enzyme that catalyzes IS movement. ISs are the smallest and simplest autonomous mobile genetic elements that contribute massively to HGT and have an important role in genome organization and evolution. Many ISs are delimited by short terminal inverted repeat (IR) and are flanked by direct repeat (DR). More than 3500 ISs from bacteria and archaea have been described. These DNA segments are capable of transposing within and between prokaryotic genomes causing insertional mutations and chromosomal rearrangements.

They cause gene inactivation and have strong polar effects or activation or alteration of the expression of adjacent genes [14–17].

Although IS elements are genomics parasites that harm their host by increasing the rate of deleterious mutations, they generate beneficial mutations trough their transposition and recombination. Indeed, IS elements are considered important elements for the adaptive evolution of their host [15, 18].

2.1.1.2. Genomic islands (GEIs)

There exists several ways how bacterial genomes can evolve, including mutations, rearrangements or HGT, contributing to diversification, and adaptation of microorganisms to environmental niches. GEIs are large DNA sequences specifically present in the genomes of certain bacteria strains but not in the genomes of closely related variants. These are non-self-mobilizing integrative and excisive elements that encode diverse functional characteristics; usually, they are integrated in bacterial chromosome but also can be found in plasmids or phages [11]. Recent information on GEIs suggests that these elements have become strongly selective for adaptive and auxiliary functions (pathogenicity, symbiosis, aromatic compound metabolism, mercury resistance, and siderophore synthesis) [19–21].

2.1.1.3. *Pathogenicity islands (PAIs)*

PAIs are a group of GEIs that carry one or more virulence-associated genes and mobility genes and occupy chromosome regions as large as 10 kb to more than 100 kb; "pathogenicity islets" are smaller fragments of DNA ranging from 1 to 10 kb. PAIs are part of a flexible gene pool that contain mobility genes so that they can be integrated into the host genome including genes encoding to integrases, transposases, phage genes, and origins of replication [22]. **Table 1** shows the main features of PAIs.

Virulence factors (VFs) are encoded by genes found in pathogenic microorganisms. Pathogenic bacteria possess various VFs that allow them colonize a variety of niches, cause infection, and survive in the hosts [23]. In order to combat infectious diseases, it is absolutely necessary to discover virulence factors of pathogenic microbes to identify targets for novel drugs and design of new vaccines [24].

A special interest has emerged on VFs study, mainly due to the constant and persistent antimicrobial resistance observed in pathogenic microorganisms, because they have modified

Genomic Islands	**Ref.**
Large segments of DNA, 10-200 kb	[22]
GC content different from the rest of the chromosome	[23]
Often inserted at tRNA genes	[23]
Usually flanked by 16-20 bp perfect or almost perfect Direct Repeats (DR)	[23]
Contain genes encoding integrases or factors related to plasmid conjugation or phages involved in GEI transfer	[23]
Often carry Insertion Elements or transposons to mobilize genetic material	[24]
Offer a selective advantage for hos bacteria and often described as pathogenicity, symbiosis, metabolic, fitness or resistance islands	[23]
Pathogenicity Islands	
Clusters of contiguous genes present in some related strains or species, but absent in non-pathogenic bacteria.	[4]
They confer on the host bacterium a complex and distinctive virulence phenotype by the presence of virulence factors.	[4]
Presence of mobility genes (integrases, transposases)	[5]
High percentage of hypothetic proteins	[5]
Different genomic sequence signature	[5]

Table 1. Characteristics of genomic and pathogenicity islands.

their virulence mechanisms to adapt to host defense system [9]. Today, complete genome sequences of different microbial species either pathogenic or non-pathogenic enable comparative studies to identify specific VFs in species through bioinformatics analyses.

As in other bacteria of clinical importance, some MGE have been identified in farm animals' pathogens. The intraerythrocytic parasite of cattle *B. bovis* has mechanisms to protect their cytoadhesion from the host adaptive immune response, and this function is mainly accomplished through antigenic variation of a virulence factor called VESA1 protein (Variant Erythrocyte Surface Antigen-1) [25]. VESA1 is a size-polymorphic, heterodimeric protein that comprises of two subunits of 105–115 and 120–135 kDa in mass approximately, depending on the isolate and clonal line [26]. Genomic and transcriptomic analyses reveal that sMORF could have a significant role for a rapid antigenic variation. However, experimental evidence is necessary [27].

In *F. hepatica,* some proteins are virulence-associated factors. These proteins are cathepsin L cysteine peptidase (FhCL) and have functions in parasite virulence including tissue invasion and suppression of host immune responses. Among the functions are degradation of red blood cells, a vital process when the parasite is located in the bile duct and needs to digest a large quantity of host cells to support the enormous production of progeny (30–50,000 eggs/day/worm) [28]. Through phylogenetic analyses, Robinson et al. [28] classified cathepsin L gene family into three clades (Clades 1, 2, and 5) expressed by tissue-migrating adult worms and two clades (Clades 3 and 4) expressed by early infective juvenile stage. Each of these cathepsins is expressed in different larvae stages. Collagenolytic activities have been reported in FhCL2 and FhCl3, suggesting that this activity is essential to the parasite in order to degrade the connective tissue matrix of the organs that break through during migration [29].

In Gram-negative pathogens, type IV Secretion System (T4SS) has a conserved structured and function that is crucial for virulence and intracellular survival. The importance of this system in *Anaplasmataceae* is its possibility as functional virulence factors due to its retention and protein conservation among rickettsial species [30]. Recently, the high complexity of the Rickettsia T4SS was revealed. Gillespie et al. [31] focus on the components of the Rickettsiales vir homolog (rvh), a collection of VirB and VirD protein-encoding genes. They found that these genes are comprised of unprecedented gene family expansion. Three families of gene duplication are contained in rvh genes: rvhb9, rvhB8, and rvhB4, and some genes are equivalent in other T4SS. This study shows the need to characterize Rickettsia rvh components.

Some molecules have been investigated because of their physiological importance in microorganisms. Aminopeptidases have been used as therapeutic and prophylactic targets in many parasitic infections and other diseases [32]. In *B. bovis,* a member of the methionine aminopeptidase (MAP) family was characterized and expressed in *E. coli*. The results showed that the construction aminopeptidase (MAP)-glutatione-S-tranferase (GST) was antigenic by inducing high levels of cytokines and immunoglobulin IgG titers in the host, and importantly, inhibitors of MAP inhibit the growth of *Babesia* parasites both *in vitro* and *in vivo* [32]. Methionine aminopeptidases have an important role in N-terminal methionine excision from the polypeptide in ribosome during protein synthesis; their physiological importance relies on the lethality of its absence in bacteria and yeast [33, 34]. MAPs in malaria play an important role in parasite biology due to their role in parasite hemoglobin during peptide catabolism [35].

Database	Website	Information	Ref.
VFDB Virulence Factor Database	http://www.mgc.ac.cn/VFs/	Curating information about virulence factors of bacterial pathogens	[33]
PAIDB v2.0 Pathogenicity Islands Database	http://www.paidb.re.kr	Pathogenicity islands (PAIs), candidate PAIs and resistance islands (REIs) in prokaryotic genomes.	[35]
PHIDIAS-Pathogen-Host Interaction Data Integration and Analysis System	http://www.phidias.us/victors/intro.php	Comprises genes experimentally observed to be necessary for virulence, including bacteria, viruses, parasites, and fungi.	[39]
MvirDB	http://mvirdb.llnl.gov/	Microbial database of protein toxins, virulence factors, and antibiotic resistance genes	[34]
PIPS Pathogenicity Island Prediction Software	http://www.bioinformatics.org/groups/?group_id=1063	Prediction of pathogenicity islands in an integrative manner.	[40]
PredictBias	http://www.bioinformatics.org/sachbinfo/predictbias.html	Identification of genomic and pathogenicity	[41]
MP3 Software	http://metagenomics.iiserb.ac.in/mp3/index.php.	Prediction of pathogenic proteins in genomic and metagenomic data	[42]
ProtVirB	http://bioinfo.icgeb.res.in/protvirdb	Database of protozoan virulent proteins	[43]
GIPSy Genomic Island Prediction Software	http://www.bioinformatics.org/groups/?group_id=1180	Prediction of GEIs including PAIs, REIs, and Symbiotic Islands (SIs)	[40]
Island Viewer 3	http://www.pathogenomics.sfu.ca/islandviewer/	Web-base resource for the prediction and analysis of GIs in bacterial and archaeal genomes	[44]
OASIS Optimized Annotation System for Insertion Sequences	https://github.com/dgrtwo/OASIS	Program that uses a library of IS to identify IS in bacteria	[45]
ISfinder	http://www-is.biotoul.fr/	Database for bacterial IS	[46]
ISsaga	http://issaga.biotoul.fr/ISsaga/issaga_index.php	Web application. Computational tools and methods for high quality IS annotation	[17]
ISQuest Software	https://omictools.com/isquest-tool	Identifies bacterial IS elements in raw read data or contigs	[47]

Table 2. Selection of online resources for analysis and search of virulence factors, toxins, GEIs, and PAIs in microorganisms [39–47].

2.2. Bioinformatics tools in pathogenomics

As mentioned before, despite the recent advances of modern medicine based on genomic data, still infectious diseases are considered as one of the biggest threats to public and animal health [36]. Comparative genomic analysis of pathogenic and non-pathogenic bacteria can reveal horizontally transferred genes between bacteria, thus conferring new properties. PAIs have some detectable properties, like genomic signatures and mobility genes helping in integration into the host genome, as genomic signatures helps to identify pathogens, functional signatures provide information about what a pathogen is capable of [5, 37].

Recently, an updated database has been reported, the Virulence Factor Database or VFDB (http://www.mgc.ac.cn/VFs/) that provide the latest information about virulence factors of various bacterial pathogens, especially those obtained by next generation sequencing technologies (NGS) [36]. The Pathogenicity Islands Database, PAIDB (http://www.paidb.re.kr), is a database that contains comprehensive information on all reported PAIs and candidate PAIs in prokaryotic genomes; additionally, information of Resistance Islands (REIs) is considered.

The importance of PAIs, a subset of GIs, is that genomes of pathogenic bacteria mediate the horizontal transfer of genes encoding a significant number of virulence factors [38].

PAIDB also contains information of antimicrobial resistance islands, REIs. This, another, class of GIs is linked to pathogenesis by conferring resistance to multiple antibiotics and thus facilitating the emergence of multidrug–resistance pathogens. PAIDB contain 223 types of PAIs and 1331 GenBank accessions of complete or partial PAI and 88 types of REIs from 108 accessions [38]. Several database and software are available for *in silico* analysis of PAIs, VFs, and IS (**Table 2**).

3. Methods used to identify pathogens

3.1. Staining and microscopic methods

Many methods are available to identify bacteria, and microscopy has an important role in microorganism identification. Especially, when an urgent diagnosis is required, fast microscopic methods are the first option. Many bacterial pathogens are identified by staining methods, and among these, differential stains are common in microbiology and provide some information about the species and many times can be compared to automated species differentiation methods [48].

Gram-stain is an old differential technique, but very popular to distinguish between Gram-positive and Gram-negative bacteria. This method is based on the different cell wall structures and components of both bacteria types. The bacterial cell wall of Gram-positives is stained by crystal violet and iodine, which form an insoluble blue dye complex while Gram-negatives are counterstained by fuchsin or safranin. This staining is also applied to some fungi, such as *Candida* spp., *Nocardia* spp., or *Actinomyces* spp. When cells walls are damaged or even cells are dead, false Gram-negatives may result [48, 49].

Another common technique is Giemsa staining, which was primarily developed for the visualization and histopathological diagnosis of *Plasmodium* spp. at the end of nineteenth century. Now, this staining method is used to identify many other parasites including *Babesia bovis, B. bigemina; Leishmania* spp., *Trypanosoma* spp.; *Toxoplasma gondii*, and others, and bacteria as *Anaplasma marginale, A. phagocytophilum*, and fungi (**Figure 2**).

The Giemsa's solution is a composition of methylene blue and oxidation products of methylene blue (Azure A and B) that stain primary proteins and nucleic acids [48].

Even natural herbal dyes as curcuma, alizarin, and henna have been used to stain *Fasciola hepatica* without the carcinogenic effect of traditional synthetic dyes [50, 51]. Fluorescent dyes such SYBR Green 1, YOYO-1, and ethidium homodimer-2 could be detected using fluorescent microscopy in combination with Giemsa staining, this method has been proposed to improve microscopic diagnosis of *Plasmodium falciparum* [52]. According to these results, the combinations of fluorescent and non-fluorescent dyes could be applied to enhance other microorganisms' identification.

Oocysts parasites identification is an issue that has been resolved through microscopic observation. In avian coccidiosis, most of the oocysts have a very similar morphological appearance with size differences that allow distinguish them. Castañón et al. [53] reported an approach based on image recognition by algorithms to identify *Eimeria* spp. oocysts; the authors extracted morphological information by using computer vision techniques in order to perform an automatic species differentiation of oocysts. The parameters considered in the identification process were: (1) multiscale curvature, (2) geometry, and, (3) texture to construct a 13-dimensional future vector for each oocyst image. With this powerful tool, molecular diagnosis based on PCR using the ribosomal ITS1 or multiplex PCR can be complemented with the use of the *Eimeria* Image Database [53].

With the recent development of fluorescent techniques and imaging tools, farm animals' pathogen identification has become a more efficient and reliable process.

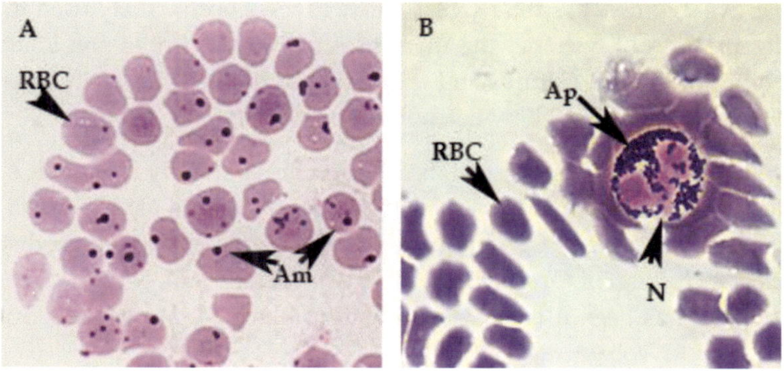

Figure 2. Visualization of (A) Giemsa staining of *A. marginale* (Am) inside bovine red blood cells (RBC), (B) Giemsa staining of *A. phagocytophylum* (Ap) inside a human neutrophil (N). (Anaplasmosis Unit, CENID-PAVET, INIFAP, Human blood was obtained with patient's consent).

3.2. Genotypic methods

Conventionally, cultural and biochemical techniques are the primary methodology for identifying most pathogens; however, Koch's postulates are critical for fulfilling most of the times [2, 54]. The culture-based testing usually yield results in several days or even up to weeks after sampling without success guaranteed, because of the unsuitable culturing conditions and the special requirements for the bacterial species [55].

Besides, pathogen identification can be a hard task when these cannot be cultured. With the development of molecular techniques and sequencing technologies, many non-cultured microorganisms, as *Mycoplasma haemobos* and *M. wenyonii* have been identified and many microorganisms already known have been reorganized phylogenetically [56].

3.2.1. Polymerase chain reaction (PCR)

Molecular methods based on nucleic acid amplification have circumvented the culturing problem with some benefits. In the molecular detection by PCR, the pathogen is first detected by PCR product amplification and then identified by sequencing, resulting in more rapid diagnoses [55]. Several pathogens of veterinary importance have been detected successfully by PCR, including *A. marginale, B. bovis, Mycobacteria* spp., *F. hepatica,* and *F. gigantica, Theileria* spp., among others [57–61]. Ribosomal RNA (rRNA) genes have emerged as the most prominent target in microbial detection mainly due to fact that the region represents a versatile mix of highly conserved and moderately to highly variable segments [62]. In bacteria, the rRNA genes are firstly transcribed from the ribosomal operon as 30S rRNA and then cleaved into 16S, 23S, and 5S rRNA by RNase III. The ribosomal operon size, nucleotide sequences, and secondary structures of 16S, 23S, and 5D rRNA are well conserved within bacterial species [63]. Since rRNA genes are evolving more slowly than protein encoding genes they have a particular importance for identification and phylogenetic analysis of distant related species [64].

3.2.1.1. Molecular markers

During the last two decades, the 16S rRNA sequences have been widely used for the identification and classification of bacteria, the main uses of 16S sequences are: identification and classification of isolated pure cultures and estimation of bacterial diversity in environmental samples without culturing through metagenomic approaches [65].

The rRNA operon in bacteria comprises 16S, 23S, and 5S, spaced by intergenic spacer regions (ITS, also called internal transcribed spacer) which have been used also to detect and differentiate pathogens [62]. Amplified PCRs products based on ITS sequences have distinguished 55 bacterial species, including 18 *Clostridium* and 15 *Mycoplasma* [66]. More recently, rRNA ITS, specifically 16S–23S, has been used in *Vibrio* identification [67], *Mycoplasma* from cattle [68], *Brucella* [69, 70], and Mycobacteria [71, 72].

Similarly to 16S rRNA, 18 s rRNA is a sequence commonly used for eukaryotic identification, such as parasites. Actually, there exists several molecular markers used to identify *B. bovis* and *B. bigemina* using 18S rRNA, cytochrome b gene, antigenic protein encoding genes msa-1 and msa-2, EF-1a, beta-tubulin, among others [73].

Alternatively, other genes less commonly used that can help in bacterial identification are chaperonin-60 (*cpn60*) [74], chaperonine GroEl [75], recombination and repair protein (*recN*), and DNA polymerase III subunits γ, τ (*dnaX*) [76], the β-subunit of RNA polymerase (*rpoB*) [76], and esterase (*est*) [77]. Among all genes used to identify bacteria, still 16S rRNA is the most used when the bacterial pathogen is non culturable, this is mostly because there exists a significant number of 16S rRNA sequences available in databases that can be used to compare and then identify [Ribosomal Database Project (http://rdp.cme.msu.edu) and Greengenes (http://greengenes.lbl.gov)]. These databases are not always complete because 16S rRNA sequences are constantly reported and many are still missing, besides, many times the species can only be identified at genus level and analyses with other genes are necessary [78].

Amplification of 16S sequence have allowed identification and phylogenetic reconstruction of several *Anaplasma* species in China, including *A. marginale y A. ovis* [79]; a comparison between *A. marginale* and *A. centrale* 16S rRNA revealed that both sequences have 98.08% identity, even with this level of identity *A. centrale* was identified by PCR primers based on 16S rRNA [80]. Bovine hemoplasmas "*Candidatus* Mycoplasma haemobos" and *Mycoplasma wenyonii* has also been detected by 16S rRNA PCR and RT-PCR in Brazil and Switzerland [81–83]. Detection of rickettsia *A. marginale*, causal agent of bovine anaplasmosis, using genomic DNA as template for PCR is an alternative diagnostic tool. Singh et al. [84] used a semi-nested PCR assay for the detection of *A. marginale* in carrier cattle in India. The PCR was optimized to identify the major surface protein 5 (Msp5) based on primers previously reported [85]. The nested PCR (nPCR) employing *msp5* primer sequences were able to detect as few as 30 infected erythrocytes per ml of the blood and then detect low levels of rickettsiaemia in cattle [85].

Noaman and Shayan [86] employed 16S ribosomal RNA (rRNA, GenBank M60313) gene of *A. marginale* on DNA isolated from blood samples of cattle. The nucleotide sequence of 16S rRNA is highly conserved in *Anaplasma* spp., and is use to amplify fragments of the gene in all known *Anaplasma* species.

B. bigemina, one of the several *Babesia* species known to cause bovine babesiosis has also been detected by PCR, besides, the amplified product is parasite and species specific [87]. From sensitivity studies, the authors showed that the 278-bp fragment amplified by PCR and visualized in reactions could contain as little as 10 pg. of parasite template DNA.

3.3. Multiplex PCR

A variant of the PCR is the multiplex PCR (mPCR) that detects more than one species at a time in a very effective way using a mixture of locus-specific primers in a single reaction [88]. mPCR offers an important advantage over single-species PCR because co-infections can be detected, for instance, detection of swine, avian and equine viruses [89–91], bacteria in fish [92], cattle bacteria and parasites, including *Mycobacterium bovis*, *T. annulata*, *F. hepatica*, and *B. bovis* [93–97], and nematodes [98] have been reported.

Multiplex PCR for detecting multiple pathogens has not been widely used in animal health diagnostic laboratories because this assay is difficult to optimize and validate [2].

3.4. PCR-restriction fragment length polymorphism (PCR-RFLP)

PCR-RFLP is an approach based on the fact that the genomes of closely related pathogen have variations in sequence, thus, a different length can be obtained from enzymatic digestion of a PCR fragment [99]. Due to that digested DNA represents a unique pattern, and this method offers a much greater sensitivity for the identification of pathogens, especially when culture is difficult. Using PCR-RFLP, *Theileria annulata* was identified in ticks (Ixodidae), showing that parasite has a preference for *Hyalomma anatolicum anatolicum* which suggest that its major role in transmission of parasite [100]. Identification of parasites as *Fasciola* species also employs PCR-RFLP analysis. The region between 18S and 28S (which includes ITS1, 5.8S, ITS2) of ribosomal RNA was amplified by PCR and then digested with restriction endonucleases, in this analysis, 90 *Fasciola* samples from different geographical regions were identified as *F. hepatica* or *F. gigantica* [58].

3.5. DNA microarrays

DNA microarrays are a viable platform for detection of pathogenic organisms. This detection has a cost lower than multiplex PCR and technologies like high-throughput sequencing [101]. A microarray is a miniaturized device that contains short single-stranded DNA oligonucleotides (25- to 70-mers) probes attached to a solid substrate. These probes would be complementary to segments of one or more target organism genome. El-Ashker et al. [59] identified *Babesia, Theileria,* and *Anaplasma* species in cattle using DNA microarray. This novel DNA microarray system was compared with microscopy and PCR assay for the diagnosis of bovine piroplasmosis and anaplasmosis. All samples positive by PCR for *Babesia/Theileria* spp. also were positive in the microarray analysis, which supports this technique as a valuable improvement in veterinary diagnoses. Another microarray developed for *Mycoplasma* spp. consist of probes for 55 different cattle pathogenic bacteria including *M. mycoides* subs. *Mycoides* [102]. To date, no microarray has been developed for diagnosis of bovine tick-borne diseases.

Acknowledgements

This work was supported by Project PN-CONACYT No. 248855.

Author details

Rosa Estela Quiroz-Castañeda

Address all correspondence to: quiroz.rosa@inifap.gob.mx

National Center for Disciplinary Research in Veterinary Parasitology, National Institute for Research in Forestry Agriculture and Livestock (CENID-PAVET, INIFAP), Jiutepec, Morelos, México

References

[1] Tomley FM, Shirley MW. Livestock infectious diseases and zoonoses. Philosophical Transactions of the Royal Society of London. Series B. The Royal Society. 2009;**364**(1530):2637-2642

[2] Cai HY, Caswell JL, Prescott JF. Nonculture molecular techniques for diagnosis of bacterial disease in animals: A diagnostic laboratory perspective. Veterinary Pathology. 2014;**51**(2):341-350

[3] Pareek CS, Smoczynski R, Tretyn A. Sequencing technologies and genome sequencing. Journal of Applied Genetics. 2011;**52**(4):413-435

[4] Pallen MJ, Wren BW. Bacterial pathogenomics. Nature. 2007;**449**(7164):835-842

[5] Che D, Hasan MS, Chen B. Identifying pathogenicity islands in bacterial pathogenomics using computational approaches. Pathogens (Basel, Switzerland). 2014;**3**(1):36-56

[6] Sudheesh PS, Al-Ghabshi A, Al-Mazrooei N, Al-Habsi S. Comparative pathogenomics of bacteria causing infectious diseases in fish. International Journal of Evolutionary Biology. 2012;**2012**:457264

[7] Sondgeroth KS, McElwain TF, Ueti MW, Scoles GA, Reif KE, Lau AOT. Tick passage results in enhanced attenuation of *Babesia bovis*. Infection and Immunity. 2014;**82**(10): 4426-4434. Adams JH, editor. 1752 N St., N.W., Washington, DC: American Society for Microbiology

[8] Cwiklinski K, Dalton JP, Dufresne PJ, La Course J, Williams DJL, Hodgkinson J, et al. The *Fasciola hepatica* genome: Gene duplication and polymorphism reveals adaptation to the host environment and the capacity for rapid evolution. Genome Biology. London: BioMed Central. 2015;**16**(1):71

[9] Beceiro A, Tomás M, Bou G. Antimicrobial resistance and virulence: A successful or deleterious association in the bacterial world? Clinical Microbiology Reviews. 2013; **26**(2):185-230

[10] Lehmann J, Matthias M, Vinetz J, Fouts D. Leptospiral pathogenomics. Pathogens. 2014; **3**(2):280-308

[11] Darmon E, Leach DRF. Bacterial genome instability. Microbiology and Molecular Biology Reviews. 2014;**78**(1):1-39

[12] Tobes R, Pareja E. Bacterial repetitive extragenic palindromic sequences are DNA targets for Insertion Sequence elements. BMC Genomics. 2006;**7**(1):1-12

[13] Van Melderen L. Toxin–antitoxin systems: Why so many, what for? Current Opinion in Microbiology. 2010;**13**(6):781-785

[14] Charlesworth B, Sniegowski P, Stephan W. The evolutionary dynamics of repetitive DNA in eukaryotes. Nature. 1994:215-220

[15] Schneider D, Lenski RE. Genome plasticity and the evolution of microbial genomes. Dynamics of insertion sequence elements during experimental evolution of bacteria. Research in Microbiology. 2004;**155**(5):319-327

[16] Mahillon J, Chandler M. Insertion sequences. Microbiology and Molecular Biology Reviews. 1998;**62**

[17] Varani AM, Siguier P, Gourbeyre E, Charneau V, Chandler M. ISsaga is an ensemble of web-based methods for high throughput identification and semi-automatic annotation of insertion sequences in prokaryotic genomes. Genome Biology. 2011;**12**(3):1-9

[18] Blot M. Transposable elements and adaptation of host bacteria. Genetica. 1994;**93**(1):5-12

[19] Sullivan JT, Trzebiatowski JR, Cruickshank RW, Gouzy J, Brown SD, Elliot RM, et al. Comparative sequence analysis of the symbiosis island of *Mesorhizobium loti* strain R7A. Journal of Bacteriology. United States. 2002;**184**(11):3086-3095

[20] Larbig KD, Christmann A, Johann A, Klockgether J, Hartsch T, Merkl R, et al. Gene islands integrated into tRNA(Gly) genes confer genome diversity on a *Pseudomonas aeruginosa* clone. Journal of Bacteriology. United States. 2002;**184**(23):6665-6680

[21] Gaillard M, Vallaeys T, Vorholter FJ, Minoia M, Werlen C, Sentchilo V, et al. The clc element of *Pseudomonas* sp. strain B13, a genomic island with various catabolic properties. Journal of Bacteriology. United States. 2006;**188**(5):1999-2013

[22] Gal-Mor O, Finlay BB. Pathogenicity islands: A molecular toolbox for bacterial virulence. Cellular Microbiology. 2006;**8**(11):1707-1719

[23] Yang J, Chen L, Sun L, Yu J, Jin Q. VFDB 2008 release: An enhanced web-based resource for comparative pathogenomics. Nucleic Acids Research. 2008;**36**(SUPPL. 1):539-542

[24] Wu H-J, Wang AH-J, Jennings MP. Discovery of virulence factors of pathogenic bacteria. Current Opinion in Chemical Biology. 2008;**12**(1):93-101

[25] Xiao Y-P, Al-Khedery B, Allred DR. The *Babesia bovis* VESA1 virulence factor subunit 1b is encoded by the 1β branch of the ves multigene family. Molecular and Biochemical Parasitology. 2010;**171**(2):81-88

[26] Allred DR, Hines SA, Ahrens KP. Isolate-specific parasite antigens of the *Babesia bovis*-infected erythrocyte surface. Molecular and Biochemical Parasitology. Netherlands. 1993;**60**(1):121-132

[27] Brayton KA, Lau AOT, Herndon DR, Hannick L, Kappmeyer LS, Berens SJ, et al. Genome sequence of *Babesia bovis* and comparative analysis of apicomplexan hemoprotozoa. PLOS Pathogens. United States. 2007;**3**(10):1401-1413

[28] Robinson MW, Tort JF, Lowther J, Donnelly SM, Wong E, Xu W, et al. Proteomics and phylogenetic analysis of the cathepsin L protease Family of the Helminth pathogen *Fasciola hepatica*: Expansion of a repertoire of virulence-associated factors. Molecular & Cellular Proteomics. 2008;**7**(6):1111-1123

[29] Robinson MW, Corvo I, Jones PM, George AM, Padula MP, To J, et al. Collagenolytic activities of the major secreted cathepsin L peptidases involved in the virulence of the Helminth pathogen, *Fasciola hepatica*. PLOS Neglected Tropical Diseases. Public Library of Science. 2011;**5**(4):e1012

[30] Sutten EL, Norimine J, Beare PA, Heinzen RA, Lopez JE, Morse K, et al. *Anaplasma marginale* type IV secretion system proteins VirB2, VirB7, VirB11, and VirD4 are immunogenic components of a protective bacterial membrane vaccine. Infection and Immunity. 2010;**78**(3): 1314-1325

[31] Gillespie JJ, Phan IQH, Driscoll TP, Guillotte ML, Lehman SS, Rennoll-Bankert KE, et al. The Rickettsia type IV secretion system: Unrealized complexity mired by gene family expansion. Pathogens and Disease. 2016;**74**(6):pii: ftw058

[32] Munkhjargal T, Ishizaki T, Guswanto A, Takemae H, Yokoyama N, Igarashi I. Molecular and biochemical characterization of methionine aminopeptidase of *Babesia bovis* as a potent drug target. Veterinary Parasitology. 2016;**221**:14-23

[33] Li X, Chang YH. Amino-terminal protein processing in *Saccharomyces cerevisiae* is an essential function that requires two distinct methionine aminopeptidases. Proceedings of the National Academy of Sciences of the United States of America. 1995;**92**(26):12357-12361

[34] Chang SY, McGary EC, Chang S. Methionine aminopeptidase gene of *Escherichia coli* is essential for cell growth. Journal of Bacteriology. United States. 1989;**171**(7):4071-4072

[35] Naughton JA, Nasizadeh S, Bell A. Downstream effects of haemoglobinase inhibition in *Plasmodium falciparum*-infected erythrocytes. Molecular and Biochemical Parasitology. Netherlands. 2010;**173**(2):81-87

[36] Chen L, Zheng D, Liu B, Yang J, Jin Q. VFDB 2016: Hierarchical and refined dataset for big data analysis—10 years on. Nucleic Acids Research. 2016;**44**(D1):D694-D697

[37] Zhou CE, Smith J, Lam M, Zemla A, Dyer MD, Slezak T. MvirDB—A microbial database of protein toxins, virulence factors and antibiotic resistance genes for bio-defence applications. Nucleic Acids Research. Oxford University Press. 2007;**35**(Database issue):D391-D394

[38] Yoon SH, Park Y-K, Kim JF. PAIDB v2.0: Exploration and analysis of pathogenicity and resistance islands. Nucleic Acids Research. 2014;**21**

[39] Xiang Z, Tian Y, He Y. PHIDIAS: A pathogen-host interaction data integration and analysis system. Genome Biology. 2007;**8**(7):1-15

[40] Soares SC, Abreu VAC, Ramos RTJ, Cerdeira L, Silva A, Baumbach J, et al. PIPS: Pathogenicity Island Prediction Software. PLoS One. Public Library of Science. 2012;**7**(2):e30848

[41] Pundhir S, Vijayvargiya HKA. PredictBias: A server for the identification of genomic and pathogenicity islands in prokaryotes. In Silico Biology. 2008;**8**(3–4):223-234

[42] Gupta A, Kapil R, Dhakan DB, Sharma VK. MP3: A software tool for the prediction of pathogenic proteins in genomic and metagenomic data. PLoS One. Public Library of Science. 2014;**9**(4):e93907

[43] Ramana J, Gupta D. ProtVirDB: A database of protozoan virulent proteins. Bioinformatics. 2009;**25**(12):1568-1569

[44] Dhillon BK, Laird MR, Shay JA, Winsor GL, Lo R, Nizam F, et al. IslandViewer 3: More flexible, interactive genomic island discovery, visualization and analysis. Nucleic Acids Research. 2015;**43**(W1):W104-W108

[45] Robinson DG, Lee M-C, Marx CJ. OASIS: An automated program for global investigation of bacterial and archaeal insertion sequences. Nucleic Acids Research. 2012;**40**(22):e174

[46] Siguier P, Perochon J, Lestrade L, Mahillon J, Chandler M. ISfinder: The reference centre for bacterial insertion sequences. Nucleic Acids Research. 2006;**34**(Suppl. 1):D32-D36

[47] Biswas A, Gauthier DT, Ranjan D, Zubair M. ISQuest: Finding insertion sequences in prokaryotic sequence fragment data. Bioinformatics. 2015;**31**(21):3406-3412

[48] Makarewicz O, Stein C, Pfister W, Loffler B, Pletz M. Identification methods—An overview. In: Popp J, Bauer M, editors. Modern Techniques for Pathogen Detection. Jena, Germany: Wiley Blacwell; 2015. p. 350

[49] Beveridge TJ. Use of the Gram stain in microbiology. Biotechnic & Histochemistry. Taylor & Francis. 2001;**76**(3):111-118

[50] Daryani A, Sharif M, Meigouni M. Staining of *Fasciola hepatica* by natural herbal dyes. Comparative Clinical Pathology. 2011;**20**(4):305-308

[51] OIE. Bovine anaplasmosis. In: OIE WO for AH, editor. OIE Terrestrial Manual 2015. OIE, World Organisation for Animal Health; 2015. Chapter 2.4.1, pp. 1-15

[52] Guy R, Liu P, Pennefather P, Crandall I. The use of fluorescence enhancement to improve the microscopic diagnosis of Falciparum malaria. Malaria Journal. 2007;**6**(1):1-8

[53] Castañón CAB, Fraga JS, Fernandez S, Gruber A, da F. Costa L. Biological shape characterization for automatic image recognition and diagnosis of protozoan parasites of the genus *Eimeria*. Pattern Recognition. 2007;**40**(7):1899-1910

[54] Cheng C, Sun J, Zheng F, Wu K, Rui Y. Molecular identification of clinical "difficult-to-identify" microbes from sequencing 16S ribosomal DNA and internal transcribed spacer 2. Annals of Clinical Microbiology and Antimicrobials. 2014;**13**(1):1

[55] Järvinen A-K, Laakso S, Piiparinen P, Aittakorpi A, Lindfors M, Huopaniemi L, et al. Rapid identification of bacterial pathogens using a PCR- and microarray-based assay. BMC Microbiology. 2009;**9**:161

[56] Martínez-Ocampo F, Rodríguez-Camarillo SD, Amaro-Estrada I, Quiroz-Castañeda RE. Draft genome sequence of "*Candidatus* Mycoplasma haemobos," a hemotropic mycoplasma identified in cattle in Mexico. Genome Announcements. 2016;**4**(4):e00656-16

[57] Figueroa JV, Chieves LP, Johnson GS, Buening GM. Multiplex polymerase chain reaction based assay for the detection of *Babesia bigemina*, *Babesia bovis* and *Anaplasma marginale* DNA in bovine blood. Veterinary Parasitology. 1993;**50**(1):69-81

[58] Mahami-Oskouei M, Dalimi A, Forouzandeh-Moghadam M, Rokni M. Molecular identification and differentiation of Fasciola isolates using PCR-RFLP method based on internal transcribed spacer (ITS1, 5.8S rDNA, ITS2). Iranian Journal of Parasitology. 2011;**6**(3):35-42

[59] El-Ashker M, Hotzel H, Gwida M, El-Beskawy M, Silaghi C, Tomaso H. Molecular biological identification of *Babesia*, *Theileria*, and *Anaplasma* species in cattle in Egypt using PCR assays, gene sequence analysis and a novel DNA microarray. Veterinary Parasitology. Elsevier BV. 2015;**207**(3–4):329-334

[60] Lopez JE, Palmer GH, Brayton KA, Dark MJ, Leach SE, Brown WC. Immunogenicity of *Anaplasma marginale* Type IV secretion system proteins in a protective outer membrane vaccine. Infection and Immunity. American Society for Microbiology. 2007;**75**(5, 5):2333-2342

[61] Carelli G, Decaro N, Lorusso a, Elia G, Lorusso E, Mari V, et al. Detection and quantification of *Anaplasma marginale* DNA in blood samples of cattle by real-time PCR. Veterinary Microbiology. 2007;**124**(1–2):107-114

[62] Sachse K. PCR detection of microbial pathogens: Specificity and performance of Diagnostic PCR assays. In: Methods in Molecular Biology. Vol. 126. Totowa, New Jersey, USA: Humana Press; 2012. pp. 3-29

[63] Maidak BL, Cole JR, Lilburn TG, Parker CT, Saxman PR, Farris RJ, et al. The RDP-II (ribosomal database project). Nucleic Acids Research. Oxford, UK: Oxford University Press. 2001;**29**(1, 1):173-174

[64] Srinivasan R, Karaoz U, Volegova M, MacKichan J, Kato-Maeda M, Miller S, et al. Use of 16S rRNA gene for identification of a broad range of clinically relevant bacterial pathogens. PLoS One. Public Library of Science. 2015;**10**(2):e0117617

[65] Rajendhran J, Gunasekaran P. Microbial phylogeny and diversity: Small subunit ribosomal RNA sequence analysis and beyond. Microbiological Research. 2011;**166**(2): 99-110

[66] Scheinert P, Krausse R, Ullmann U, Söller R, Krupp G. Molecular differentiation of bacteria by PCR amplification of the 16S–23S rRNA spacer. Journal of Microbiological Methods. 1996;**26**(1):103-117

[67] Hoffmann M, Brown EW, Feng PCH, Keys CE, Fischer M, Monday SR. PCR-based method for targeting 16S-23S rRNA intergenic spacer regions among *Vibrio* species. BMC Microbiology. 2010;**10**(1):1-14

[68] Tamiozzo PJ, Estanguet AA, Maito J, Tirante L, Pol M, Giraudo JA. Detection of *Mycoplasma canadense* and *Mycoplasma californicum* in dairy cattle from Argentina. Revista Argentina de Microbiologia. 2014;**46**(2):119-121

[69] Yu WL, Nielsen K. Review of Detection of Brucella sp. by Polymerase Chain Reaction. Croatian Medical Journal. Croatian Medical Schools. 2010;**51**(4):306-313

[70] Rijpens NP, Jannes G, Van Asbroeck M, Rossau R, Herman LM. Direct detection of *Brucella* spp. in raw milk by PCR and reverse hybridization with 16S-23S rRNA spacer probes. Applied and Environmental Microbiology. 1996;**62**(5):1683-1688

[71] Park H, Jang H, Kim C, Chung B, Chang CL, Park SK, et al. Detection and identification of mycobacteria by amplification of the internal transcribed spacer regions with genus- and species-specific PCR primers. Journal of Clinical Microbiology. American Society for Microbiology. 2000;**38**(11):4080-4085

[72] Sevilla IA, Molina E, Elguezabal N, Pérez V, Garrido JM, Juste RA. Detection of mycobacteria, *Mycobacterium avium* subspecies, and *Mycobacterium tuberculosis* complex by a novel tetraplex real-time PCR assay. Journal of Clinical Microbiology. 2015;**53**(3): 930-940

[73] Ríos TS, Ríos OL. Principal molecular markers used to identify *Babesia bovis* and *Babesia bigemina*. Revista MVZ Córdoba. Universidad de Córdoba, Montería, Colombia. 2011;**16** (2):2470-2483

[74] Links MG, Dumonceaux TJ, Hemmingsen SM, Hill JE. The chaperonin-60 universal target is a barcode for bacteria that enables *de novo* assembly of metagenomic sequence data. PLoS One. Public Library of Science. 2012;**7**(11):1-10

[75] Ybañez AP, Sivakumar T, Battsetseg B, Battur B, Altangerel K, Matsumoto K, et al. Specific molecular detection and characterization of *Anaplasma marginale* in Mongolian cattle. The Journal of Veterinary Medical Science. 2013;**75**(4):399-406

[76] Zeigler DR. Gene sequences useful for predicting relatedness of whole genomes in bacteria. International Journal of Systematic and Evolutionary Microbiology. 2003;**53**(6): 1893-1900

[77] Miranda KR, Neves FPG, dos Santos-Filho J, de Paula GR, Lobo LA, Oelemann WMR, et al. Application of DNA sequence analysis based on five different conserved genes (16S rDNA, rpoB, gdh, est and pgm) for intra-species discrimination of *Bacteroides fragilis*. Anaerobe. 2013;**19**:58-61

[78] Yarza P, Spröer C, Swiderski J, Mrotzek N, Spring S, Tindall BJ, et al. Sequencing orphan species initiative (SOS): Filling the gaps in the 16S rRNA gene sequence database for all species with validly published names. Systematic and Applied Microbiology. 2013;**36**(1):69-73

[79] Liu Z, Luo J, Bai Q, Ma M, Guan G, Yin H. Amplification of 16S rRNA genes of *Anaplasma* species in China for phylogenetic analysis. Veterinary Microbiology. 2005; **107**(1–2):145-148

[80] Inokuma H, Terada Y, Kamio T, Raoult D, Brouqui P. Analysis of the 16S rRNA gene sequence of *Anaplasma centrale* and Its phylogenetic relatedness to other *Ehrlichiae*.

Clinical and Diagnostic Laboratory Immunology. American Society for Microbiology. 2001;**8**(2):241-244

[81] Girotto A, Zangirolamo AF, Bogado ALG, Souza ASLE, da Silva GCF, Garcia JL, et al. Molecular detection and occurrence of "*Candidatus* Mycoplasma haemobos" in dairy cattle of Southern Brazil. Revista Brasileira de Parasitologia Veterinária. 2012;**21**(3):342-344

[82] Meli ML, Willi B, Dreher UM, Cattori V, Knubben-Schweizer G, Nuss K, et al. Identification, molecular characterization, and occurrence of two bovine hemoplasma species in Swiss cattle and development of real-time TaqMan quantitative PCR assays for diagnosis of bovine hemoplasma infections. Journal of Clinical Microbiology. 2010; **48**(10):3563-3568

[83] McAuliffe L, Lawes J, Bell S, Barlow A, Ayling R, Nicholas R. The detection of *Mycoplasma* (formerly *Eperythrozoon*) *wenyonii* by 16S rDNA PCR and denaturing gradient gel electrophoresis. Veterinary Microbiology. 2006;**117**(2–4):292-296

[84] Singh H, Jyoti HM, Singh NK, Rath SS. Molecular detection of *Anaplasma marginale* infection in carrier cattle. Ticks and Tick-Borne Diseases. Elsevier GmbH. 2012;**3**(1):55-58

[85] Torioni de Echaide S, Knowles DP, McGuire TC, Palmer GH, Suarez CE, McElwain TF. Detection of cattle naturally infected with *Anaplasma marginale* in a region of endemicity by nested PCR and a competitive enzyme-linked immunosorbent assay using recombinant major surface protein 5. Journal of Clinical Microbiology. American Society for Microbiology. 1998;**36**(3):777-782

[86] Noaman V, Shayan P. Comparison of microscopy and PCR-RFLP for detection of *Anaplasma marginale* in carrier cattle. Iranian Journal of Microbiology. Tehran University of Medical Sciences. 2010;**2**(2):89-94

[87] Figueroa JV, Chieves LP, Johnson GS, Buening GM. Detection of *Babesia bigemina*-infected carriers by polymerase chain reaction amplification. Journal of Clinical Microbiology. 1992;**30**(10):2576-2582

[88] Markoulatos P, Siafakas N, Moncany M. Multiplex polymerase chain reaction: A practical approach. Journal of Clinical Laboratory Analysis. John Wiley & Sons, Inc. 2002; **16**(1):47-51

[89] Lee E, Kim E-J, Shin Y-K, Song J-Y. Design and testing of multiplex RT-PCR primers for the rapid detection of influenza A virus genomic segments: Application to equine influenza virus. Journal of Virological Methods. 2016;**228**:114-122

[90] Zeng Z, Liu Z, Wang W, Tang D, Liang H, Liu Z. Establishment and application of a multiplex PCR for rapid and simultaneous detection of six viruses in swine. Journal of Virological Methods. 2014;**208**:102-106

[91] Yao LN, Ruan W, Zeng CY, Li ZH, Zhang X, Lei YL, et al. Pathogen identification and clinical diagnosis for one case infected with *Babesia*. Chinese Journal of Parasitology & Parasitic Diseases. 2012;**30**

[92] Mata AI, Gibello A, Casamayor A, Blanco MM, Domínguez L, Fernández-Garayzábal JF. Multiplex PCR assay for detection of bacterial pathogens associated with warm-water Streptococcosis in Fish. Applied and Environmental Microbiology. American Society for Microbiology. 2004;**70**(5):3183-3187

[93] Picozzi K, Carrington M, Welburn SC. A multiplex PCR that discriminates between *Trypanosoma brucei brucei* and zoonotic *T. b. rhodesiense*. Experimental Parasitology. 2008; **118**(1):41-46

[94] Santín M, Zarlenga DS. A multiplex polymerase chain reaction assay to simultaneously distinguish *Cryptosporidium* species of veterinary and public health concern in cattle. Veterinary Parasitology. 2009;**166**(1–2):32-37

[95] Junlong L, Li Y, Liu A, Guan G, Xie J, Yin H, et al. Development of a multiplex PCR assay for detection and discrimination of *Theileria annulata* and *Theileria sergenti* in cattle. Parasitology Research. 2015;**114**(7):2715-2721

[96] Araujo CP, Osorio ALAR, Jorge KSG, Ramos CAN, Filho AFS, Vidal CES, et al. Detection of *Mycobacterium bovis* in bovine and bubaline tissues using nested-PCR for TbD1. PLoS One. Public Library of Science. 2014;**9**(3):e91023

[97] Bilgiç HB, Karagenç T, Simuunza M, Shiels B, Tait A, Eren H, et al. Development of a multiplex PCR assay for simultaneous detection of *Theileria annulata, Babesia bovis* and *Anaplasma marginale* in cattle. Experimental Parasitology. 2013;**133**(2):222-229

[98] Zarlenga DS, Barry Chute M, Gasbarre LC, Boyd PC. A multiplex PCR assay for differentiating economically important gastrointestinal nematodes of cattle. Veterinary Parasitology. 2001;**97**(3):201-211

[99] OIE WO for AH. Biotechnology in the diagnosis of infectious diseases. In: Manual for Diagnostic Test and Vaccines for Terrestrial Animals. 7th Editio ed. OIE, World Organisation for Animal Health; 2015. pp. 1322-1337

[100] Tavassoli M, Tabatabaei M, Nejad BE, Tabatabaei MH, Najafabadi A, Pourseyed SH. Detection of *Theileria annulata* by the PCR-RFLP in ticks (Acari, Ixodidae) collected from cattle in West and North-West Iran. Acta Parasitologica. 2011;**56**(1):8-13

[101] McLoughlin KS. Microarrays for pathogen detection and analysis. Briefings in Functional Genomics. 2011;**19**

[102] Tonelli A, Sacchini F, Krasteva I, Zilli K, Scacchia M, Beaurepaire C, et al. One test microbial diagnostic microarray for identification of *Mycoplasma mycoides* subsp. mycoides and other *Mycoplasma* species. Molecular Biotechnology. 2012;**52**(3):285-299

Chapter 2

Immune System and Its Relationships with Pathogens: Structure, Physiology, and Molecular Biology

Hugo Aguilar-Díaz and Raquel Cossío-Bayúgar

Additional information is available at the end of the chapter

http://dx.doi.org/10.5772/intechopen.72635

Abstract

Ticks are of vast medical and veterinary public health importance due to direct damage in livestock by its hematophagous feeding habits and its potential as a vector capable to transmit infectious agents such as Tick-borne diseases. Currently, the knowledge of vertebrates' immune system contributes to the advance in vaccine and drug development, resulting in new drugs that help to control human and livestock pathogens. Unfortunately, very small advances have been achieved in tick's immune system that could help to develop new strategies designated to control tick-borne diseases and other arthropod vectors. On this subject, the study of the mechanisms involved is transcendental as is also the study on molecules, cells, and regulation of immune response involved in signaling pathways in ticks. The progress on the understanding of ticks' physiology represents a necessary advance in molecular approaches related with a tick's immune response, involved in host-vector-pathogen interaction, and, in turn, evolutionary relationships. Current knowledge on tick's immune response to different kinds of pathogens is described in this chapter and the use of modern molecular tools to fill the gaps on different aspects in tick immunobiology that still is unclear or under study.

Keywords: ticks, immune system, pathogens, hemolymph

1. Introduction

Ixodidae, comprising those arthropods commonly called ticks, include nearly 870 acaridae species, and these are obligate hematophagous parasites of terrestrial vertebrates at some part of their life cycle. Moreover, ticks are considered as important veterinary health threat, due to their capacity to cause direct damage to livestock by feeding on blood and transmitting tick-borne pathogens, causing serious animal and human infectious diseases. The pathogenic diversity of organisms transmitted by ticks exceeds to be found in all other hematophagous arthropods. Tick-borne pathogens include protozoans, the bacteria rickettsia, viruses, and nematodes [1] that in turn evade the tick's immune defense mechanisms, encountered on their route through the tick's body (midgut, hemolymph, salivary glands or ovaries). These immune interactions are very important in tick biology and pathogen relationships. Likewise, some pathogens are also often trans-stadia and trans-ovarian transmitted increasing the vector-pathogen complexity, related with a disease transmission and severity, considering that each tick species is capable to transmit different pathogens [2]. Unfortunately, many metabolic and molecular mechanisms related with a tick's immune response to different pathogens remain unclear. For this reason, in recent years, the study of tick-host-pathogen interface has increased. Currently, we know that tick's innate immunity is carried on by the cellular and innate responses, where the different molecules, enzymes, cells, and proteins are involved in general immune mechanism. On the other hand, we have different molecular and immunological tools, as tick's salivary glands, midgut transcriptome, and proteomics analysis, and the first tick genome project, that contribute to elucidate tick's biological interactions. The immunobiology characterization of the tick-pathogen-host interface dynamic interaction should be exploited as a tool used for development of novel vector and transmission blocking vaccines, targets, and new drug design [3, 4].

2. Immune system in invertebrates

All invertebrates have an immune system, composed of both humoral and cellular response that results as effective defense to different pathogen attack. The cellular immune response is composed of several mechanisms as phagocytosis, nodulation formation, agglutination, and cellular encapsulation, while humoral response involves expression and secretion of different molecules able to kill bacteria, parasites, and other pathogens [2, 4]. The performance of this multifactorial system requires synthesis and regulation of RNA and proteins involved in arthropod protection. Until recently, the investigations of molecular, genetics, and cellular aspects of the arthropods' immune response were scant. One reason behind this paucity is the extremely difficult to control laboratory conditions that allow to maintain the host-parasite interaction in several generations, or different stages of arthropod life cycle [2]. On the other hand, among the invertebrates, the insects have received most attention, compared to arachnids. In this regard, in spite of extensive research, the immune system of ticks is still poorly understood.

2.1. Ticks' immunobiological response

The immune response of ticks as well as arthropods includes both cellular and humoral mechanisms, where the hemolymph and other tissues, such as salivary glands, midgut, hemolymph, and fat body, provide the principal source of molecules and cells involved in the immunological attack of pathogens. In the case of tick's hemolymph, many pathways involved in the immune response still remain unclear [4]. Currently, few reports explain the type of response that ticks have against different infectious agents that, in turn, could be used as target to pest biocontrol.

3. Cellular immune response

3.1. Hemolymph

All tissues in ticks, and other invertebrates, are bathed in a fluid known as the hemolymph, which is the first source of nutrients, osmoregulation, and molecules and hormones transport, and provide protection to pathogen agents to which ticks are exposed [1]. Likewise, hemolymph coagulates at the site of some injury, preventing microbes spreading into the body tissues. The hemolymph consists of protein-rich plasma and different types of cells called hemocytes that play a transcendental role in immune response [2].

3.1.1. Hemocytes

In ticks, the immune cell–mediated response is carried out by hemocytes, cells with free circulation and the major component of the hemolymph. Hemocytes play an important role in the tick's defense against injury as well as microbial infection and increase greatly its population, in response to bacteria, viruses, protozoa, and other pathogen infection; however, the multiplication rates for the hemocyte types in response to a specific pathogen have not been fully clarified [5–8]. The mature hemocytes mediate different events that include phagocytosis, nodulation, and encapsulation. The tick hemolymph can be divided into four cell types based on their function and morphology; however, at the moment, the hemocytes classification is controversial, because it has been observed that population may varied in hard and soft ticks and among species. The prohemocytes are round to oval small cells with a prominent nucleus, numerous mitochondria, and little granular cytoplasm. The cell size is 6–7 μm and represents the stem cells in the hemolymph, from which all cell types can be differentiated and occasionally can be found to be associated with many tissues. The prohemocytes' population proportion varies depending on the species and healthy, wounded, or infected ticks [9, 10]. The granulocytes are large cells with numerous cytoplasmatic granules; some cases have a cytoplasmatic extension called filopodia. In general, granulocytes have a long size about 15–20 μm and are further subdivided into type I and type II, depending on the granule morphology. Type I granulocytes are pleomorphic cells that 6 μm in length, which contain variable electrodense granules and presence of filopodia and lysosomes. The type II granulocytes contain several granules both electrodense and condensing immature granules, located peripherally and at the central cell [11]. Along with granulocytes, the plasmatocytes are the most predominant hemocyte type in hemolymph. These cells have slightly elongated shape, often fusiform and numerous filopodia, with a large variability in size ranging from 8 to 12 and the long axis up to 20 μm. In some species, plasmatocytes have rounded or ovoid shape, with a size about 10–12 μm and containing few vacuoles and granules. The spherulocytes are cells with a size of 11–14 μm and are oval shaped with electron-lucent and fibril-filled granules that fill almost the entire cytoplasm cell. Currently, some studies report the presence of the oenocytoids in limited number of tick species [10]. These cells are 11–18 μm in size and are ovoid shaped with cytoplasmatic granules [12]. However, the oenocytoids' presence in ticks remains controversial [1]. The understanding of functions and pathways involved in the activation of hemocytes could provide elements that help to understand the cells' role in immune response. In this regard, many groups have studies based on electrophoretic patterns in one and two dimension, obtaining proteomic maps that show proteins related with the hemocytes' pathogen response [13].

3.2. Phagocytosis

Phagocytosis is a complex mechanism that involves the recognition, engulfment, and destruction of pathogens. In this process, the immune cells recognize pathogen-associated molecular patterns (PAMPs) produced by several bacteria and fungi. In all arthropods, phagocytosis is carried out by the hemocytes and represents the first primary defense response to pathogen infection [11, 14]. In ticks, the phagocytosis process has been regulated by granulocytes type I and plasmocytes and sometimes by granulocytes type II, suggesting that differences in hemocytes' population have different roles and contributions to the tick's immune response [15]. In initial steps, the phagocytic cell response is binding receptor-mediated to pathogen cell surface; subsequently, signal transduction pathways are activated and followed by filopodia projections that surround and engulf the bound particle [16]. The particle is internalized by endocytosis into a vesicle, subsequently, with lysosomal compartments that in turn form the phagolysosome. Inside, intracellular enzymes are activated such as acid phosphatases, type c lysozyme, cystatins, and proteases completing the cellular lysis. Little is known about the molecular regulation in tick immune response, some reports suggested that as in insects the most important signal transduction pathways are mitogen-activated protein kinase (MAPK) and FAK/Src pathways that in turn are involved in proPO activation [16]. Moreover, several external factors are capable to enhance this process. Currently, recent evidence indicates that *R. microplus* produces reactive oxygen species (ROS)-mediated oxidative burst modulated by protein kinase C, similar to that found in leucocytes [17].

3.3. Nodulation

Tick hemocytes are capable of expressing lectins on membrane surface involved in pathogen recognition. These molecules can join with lipopolysaccharides (LPS) also present on the pathogen surface. Currently, several lectins involved in the immune response and other mechanisms have been identified in tick hemocytes and different cells [18–21]. In soft ticks, *O. moubata* was described to have a protein called Dorin-M, lectin with high hemagglutinating activity and isolated from hemocytes, and hemolymph plasma [22]; likewise, *I. ricinus* was described to have the Ixoderin A, lectin found in midgut and hemocytes [23]. The protein-carbohydrate interaction confers the ability to hemocyte aggregation that results in the pathogen entrapment and, in turn, the opsonization through lectins that may also cause bacteria aggregates [24].Thus, lectin recognition leads hemocyte recruitment that builds a sticky mass around the bacterial aggregate (nodules), preventing the dissemination of pathogens and eventually digesting it. The formation of this nodule represents a predominant cellular immunity defense mechanism to bacterial challenges [25].

3.4. Encapsulation

Encapsulation is the immunological process whereby the arthropods are capable of attacking pathogens that are very large to eliminate by nodulation or phagocytosis. Other immunological processes, such as the proteolytic degradation of microbial products (LPS and peptidoglycan), can result in the prophenoloxidase activation. This activation generates phenoloxidase expression that in turn, along with tyrosine metabolism, is directly related to melanin synthesis. In all insects, pathogen encapsulation involves melanization, where hemocytes, mainly type I granulocytes and plasmatocytes, form a capsule of thick layer around the pathogen that leads to asphyxiation and toxic-free radical production, such as quinones and semiquinones [3, 26, 27], with melanin deposition as the final step [10]. In ticks, phenoloxidase is present in *O. moubata* hemolymph [28], in contrast to *A. americanum, D. variabilis, and I. scapularis,* where there are no reports to phenoloxidase activity [29]. In this regard, in hard tick *D. variabilis,* the simple injection of plastic bead can induce the capsule formation, but without the presence of melanization [30]. These findings suggest that this pathway is present in ticks; however, it has a distinct role in metabolism or immune response. Moreover, genomic analyses in VectorBase indicate the absence of gene homologs for the complete pathway in *I. scapularis* genome sequence [31].

4. Humoral immune response

The humoral factors of the insect and crustacean immune system have been extensively studied. In contrast, in ticks, we know very little of this field. Mostly, the soluble factors are produced by hemocytes and released in the hemolymph, where they are transported to other tissues such as midgut and salivary glands. The humoral factors play an important role in the defense and protection of ticks from microbial invasion. Within these factors, a variety of antimicrobial proteins, such as lectins, proteases, and lysozymes, coagulation factors, proteases inhibitors, antimicrobial peptides, and products related to oxidative stress, are included [3, 32]. These soluble factors are involved in various aspects of the immune protection, such as blood ticks feeding in midgut protection; during migration hemolymph defense; and tissue protection, for example, during pathogen transmission in salivary glands, in all cases during pathogen infestation [2]. The plasma hemolymph represents nearly 90% of total composition, and the proteic soluble component represents approximately 11.5–14.3% of plasma [33]. The knowledge of ticks' hemolymph components is very limited; for this reason, the advance in the understanding is based on other arthropods [33]. For example, electrophoresis assays of two-dimensional gel map obtained of *Drosophila melanogaster* show 160 hemolymph proteins. The results found have been used as basis for comparative studies in other species, including ticks [34].

4.1. Antimicrobial peptides (AMPs)

Antimicrobial peptides (AMPs) represent the most effective humoral immune response, for their ability to kill several pathogens, for their fast response, and for their effectiveness at micronanomolar concentrations. AMPs are small peptides (3–20 kDa), and their action mechanism is based on their capacity to cell membrane or cell wall binding, causing structural disruption that results in loss of pathogen membrane potential. AMPs are secreted mainly by the fat body and hemocytes; however, midgut is capable to produce some peptides [2]. Many authors reported and identified several AMPs in ticks, including microplusin [35], hebraein [36], ixodidin [37], antimicrobial peptide (ISAMP) [38], and some peptides from *Amblyomma hebraeum* [39].

4.1.1. Defensins

Defensins are small cationic peptides (3–6 kDa) with six to eight cystein residues that are folded by three or four disulfide bridges. These bonds help to stabilize and maintain the tertiary structure, called "defensin folds" [40]. Defensin AMPs were found in many arthropods including hard and soft ticks [41, 42]. Defensins may be classified into three major groups: (1) peptides with α-helical conformation, (2) cyclic and open cyclic peptides with cysteine residue pairs, and (3) peptides with overrepresentation of some amino acids [3]. In all cases, the mature peptides present highly conserved regions in contrast with leader regions that show much more variability. Moreover, its sequence contains hydrophobic regions separated from charged regions that enable them to insert into pathogen membranes causing pores that in turn kill the cell [43]. In ticks, the defensin expression is carried out in several tissues such as fat body, hemocytes, salivary glands, and midgut. *In silico* genetic analysis shows the presence of two multigene families of defensin-like peptides. The first family, corresponds to scapularisin-type defensin peptides [44], and the second, the scasin defensin-like peptides, which present low similarity with other defensins; however, they have six conserved cysteine residue characteristics of defensins. Several tick species present multiple defensin isoforms, with regulation tissue-dependent expression. However, *in silico* analysis shows that the protein sequences are very closely related in mature regions. In contrast, three defensins from the hard ticks *Amblyomma hebraeum, Haemaphysalis longicornis,* and microplusin from *R. microplus* are the exception of this analysis. Defensin sequence analyses demonstrated four isoforms (A, B, C, and D) present in soft tick *O. moubata*. On the other hand, some assays with several component of bacterial wall, injected into tick´s hemolymph showed upregulation of defensin expression by semiquantitative RT-PCR and ELISA [45]. Interestingly, isoforms A, B, and C are overexpressed in midgut, while isoform D is overexpressed in fat body [46]. These results suggested that defensin isoforms are expressed in tissue-dependent fashion. However, the receptors and signaling pathways require more analysis.

4.1.2. Lysozymes

Lysozymes are ubiquitously expressed enzymes with a molecular weight approximately 14 kDa, are involved in digestive processes, and have an antimicrobial activity for their ability to lyse bacteria by hydrolyzing the β-1,4 glycosidic bonds between the N-acetyl-muramic acid and N-acetyl-D-glucosamine residues that form the peptidoglycan walls. In a hard tick *D. variabilis*, the expression of C-type lysozyme, which increases in hemolymph 17-fold, after exposition to *E. coli* at 72 h post-challenge, has been demonstrated [47]. In this case, the level of C-type lysozyme in hemolymph is highest than in midgut and other tissue [48, 49]. In contrast, C-type lysozyme (HI-lysozyme) from *H. longicornis* [50] is detected in all development stages of ticks and in gene expression in fat body, midgut, ovaries, and hemolymph and is upregulated after bacterial challenge. Likewise, the hard tick *O. moubata* expresses a 124 amino acid C-type lysozyme that presents overexpression in midgut, after blood feeding, but not in the tick hemolymph [51]. These results suggest that tick lysozyme is an enzyme with both immune and metabolic functions [51, 52]. Moreover, the lysozymes present in ticks' hemolymph may act synergistically with defensin and other AMPs in the pathogen control by disruption of bacteria cell wall, accelerating the killing action [41].

http://dx.doi.org/10.5772/intechopen.72635

4.1.3. Other antimicrobial peptides

Currently, in addition to defensins, there exist a large number of antimicrobial peptides identified. In ticks, other types of AMPs have been detected. In *R. microplus*, microplusin, a polypeptide of 10 kDa, is present in hemolymph and presents no sequence similarity with any AMP reported [35]. Structurally, the polypeptide has six cysteine residues, and the gene expression was observed in different tissues such as fat body, ovaries, and hemocytes, suggesting that the mature peptide must be released into the hemolymph. The hebraein is an 11 kDa antimicrobial protein with six cysteine residues and one histidine-rich carboxyl-terminal region. This AMP was isolated from the hemolymph of female *Amblyomma hebraeum* ticks [36]. *In silico* analysis showed similarities and identities between hebraein and microplusin of 73 and 62%, respectively, and this suggests that probably hebraein belongs to the same family and, structurally, has the cysteine motif similar to microplusin. The hebraein is a protein with widespread antimicrobial activity, experimentally demonstrated by different assays, by both recombinant and native proteins against the Gram-positive (*Staphylococcus aureus*) and Gram-negative (*E. coli*) bacteria, and in turn showed antipathogen activity against fungi [53]. Additional experiments demonstrated that histidine-deficient mutants of the protein lack antimicrobial activity. On the other hand, the Ixosin was identified in *Ixodes sinensis*, a peptide of 2.8 kDa isolated from salivary glands, described as the first antimicrobial peptide lacking cysteine residues [53]. Ixosin has an antimicrobial activity against Gram-positive and Gram-negative bacteria and fungi [53]. Additionally, a novel antimicrobial peptide was isolated from the *R. microplus* hemocytes [35]. This peptide was named ixodidin, and demonstrated inhibitory effects against *E. coli* and *Micrococcus luteus* growth [35]; in addition, ixodidin, has a proteolytic inhibitory activity against serine proteinases. This is a first report, the molecule in arachnid with both proteinase activity and bacterial growth.

4.2. Hemagglutination (lectins)

Lectins are proteins whose structure has domains with specific binding sites for carbohydrate [54]. The bacteria membrane or cell wall including the fungi and protozoan pathogens has different carbohydrate moieties that can be recognized by lectins. These proteins exhibit different molecular sizes from 30 to 85 kDa and have been identified in the membrane surface of hemocytes, cell gut, and salivary glands, or synthesized by hemocytes and released in the hemolymph plasma of soft and hard tick species. In invertebrates, lectins are important mediators of immune response. Initially, these molecules are defined by their participation in a hemagglutination process; however, these proteins also bind to pathogens that, in turn, enable hemocytes to recognize and engulf (opsonization). This process includes carbohydrate recognition by ficolins and mannose-binding gal-lectins, among others [55, 56]. Insects, ascidians, crustaceans, and ticks contain molecule type TLP-1 and TLP-2 lectins (*Tachypleustridentatus*), to form molecule clusters that bind and immobilize pathogens [10, 23, 55–57]. The mechanism causes pathogen be trapped and immobilized forming aggregates, which later are surrounded by hemocytes and destroyed by encapsulation or nodulation [58]. Tick lectins are involved in processes of cell adhesion, recognition, opsonization, phagocytosis, and cytolysis of infecting pathogens [59]. The first tick lectin reports were in the papillipes *Ornithodoros tartakovsky* and

O. tholozani [60, 61]. Subsequently, in *O. moubata* hemolymph plasma was identified the lectin Dorin M, lectin to 640 kDa, synthesized in the hemocytes and secreted into the hemolymph plasma, which has a high hemagglutinating capacity [19, 57, 62]. In this regard, molecular structure studies showed that Dorin M lectin has a fibrinogen-like domain related to the ficolin family of proteins that recognizes carbohydrate sequences, especially sialic acid and N-acetyl-D-glucosamine, similar to the tachylectins of *T. tridentatus* [57]. OMFREP is a potential lectin in *O. moubata* and has been identified in hemocytes [23]. The use of the bioinformatics approach complemented with molecular studies results in the identification of fibrinogen-related protein that presents a 65% identity and a similar tissue distribution to Dorin M [23]. Likewise, novel galectin (OmGalec) has a different tissue and stage distribution in *O. moubata* [21]. This protein has galactose-binding properties and consists of tandem repeated carbohydrate recognition domains, where the carbohydrate affinity typical motif is present [21]. In hard tick *I. ricinus*, Ixoderin A is expressed by hemocytes and is present in midgut and salivary glands, while Ixoderin B is only expressed in salivary glands. These findings suggest that the lectin and isoforms have a selective expression in different tissue, plasma, and cells, suggesting that they have specific roles; however, many pathways are still unknown. In salivary glands and the midgut of *Rhipicephalus appendiculatus* was described a lectin that was related to a significant increase of sugar, which inhibits hemagglutination during *Theileria parva* infection, suggesting a decisive role in this process [63, 64]. Recently, it was demonstrated that some lectins are involved in various processes related to feeding [65], ticks' immune cell regulation, and molecule recognition. Interestingly, the cloning and protein expression in ticks' hemocytes and salivary glands of two fibrinogen-related proteins, which present high homology with Dorin M lectin, showed that they are essential in the pathogen transmission [20].

4.3. Proteases and protease inhibitors

4.3.1. Proteases

The feeding mechanisms of ticks involve the presence of midgut, where the blood mead digestion is carried out. In this process, a large variety of cysteine, aspartic, and serine proteases are involved, and many of these molecules also have an important role in mechanisms of immune response. In the lumen, the serine proteases are the most important, which function as hemolytic agents and as cysteine and aspartyl proteases in hemoglobin digestion [66–68]. Various of these proteins are identified; however, in ticks, the regulation, expression, and presence of these molecules still remain unclear. Currently, the protease immune mechanism in insects suggests that metalloproteases may be important in cellular immune defense [69]. In the *D. variabilis* midgut, three metalloproteinases have been identified from cDNA library [70]. In this regard, analysis of sequences showed very little similarity to tick proteases, suggesting that these may be novel metalloproteinases. Likewise, a clip-domain serine proteinase homolog was identified [71]. On the other hand, the arthropod clip-domain family serine proteinases contain two major domains: a trypsin gen-like catalytic domain in the C-terminus and a disulfide knotted regulatory N-terminal domain [72]. In this regard, the *Anopheles* mosquitoes present serine protease overexpression in response to malarial parasites. This mechanism is consistent with the innate immune response generated for the hemolymph [73]. This response is a key factor in the internal control for malaria parasites' number and replication. Similarly, tick hemocytes are able to responsd with an immune-responsive factor D-like overexpression, in response to Gram-positive challenge [72]. *In silico* analysis showed that immune-responsive factor D-like overexpression has a 54% sequence identity to *Tachypleus tridentatus* serine proteases [74]. It is important to note that the similar domains present in these proteases are found in high invertebrates variety, suggesting the conservation of these molecules [72].

4.3.2. Protease inhibitors

Protease inhibitors are important in tick's pathogen infection as innate immune suppressor of virulence, toxic, and replication factors expressed by microorganisms. Proteases are important virulence factors used in various stages of the infection process, both by prokaryote and eukaryote pathogens. The inactivation of these factors may prevent the pathogen survival in the tick [75].Two major protease inhibitors have been reported in ticks: one called serpins that act as serine proteinase inhibitors and the other α-macroglobulins, large glycoproteins with mostly thiol-ester–containing proteinase inhibitors. Serpins may be found in plasma hemolymph and small cytoplasm granules [76]; however, in *R. appendiculatus* ticks, four serpins in midgut, salivary glands, and other internal tissues have been reported [67]. Moreover, in an *A. americanum* tick, a large number of serpin transcripts were described, many of which were ubiquitously expressed in the midgut (three most strongly expressed); likewise, several transcripts were also expressed in salivary glands and ovary [77]. In reference to immune response, serpins are involved in the fungal or bacterial protease inhibition and protection from several infections. Serpins, containing an active site serine replaced by glycine [47], also are involved in the regulation of several proteases that in turn contribute as cofactors in coagulation and cytokine activation and, most interesting, as a cofactor involved in prophenoloxidase pathway activation [78]. This activation suggests the phenoloxidase (PO) pathway presence in ticks, something that still is controversial. However, serpins could be an antigen target to the development of antitick vaccine or new drugs, since apparently it is related to the tick homeostasis, because of their potential functions as protease inhibitors [79]. The second proteinase inhibitor present in hemolymph ticks is the α-macroglobulins. This protease inhibitor family includes the α-2-macroglobulins, operating by neutralization of pathogen proteases by "entrapping in a molecular cage" through bait region, when protease substrate is recognized [80]. The molecular cage formation activates a proteolytic cleavage, through both the bait region and four thioester bond ruptures that in turn stabilize α-2-macroglobulin complexes, followed by the entrapment and protease transportation to hemolymph, which are degraded by lysosomes of hemocyte phagocyte cells [80]. In hard tick *I. scapularis*, cDNA sequence obtained from the salivary glands shows evidence of the α-2-macroglobulin presence, and in the soft tick *O. moubata*, α-2-macroglobulin present in hemolymph plasma is capable of inhibiting the trypsin action [81, 82]. Another important group of the cysteine protease inhibitors is the cystatins. The cystatins belong to protease family, which are reversible inhibitors of papain-like cysteine proteases, which function as proteolysis mediators, preventing the damage caused by cystein protease release to lysosome. In various species, cystatins are implicated in several functions related to immune response, epidermal homeostasis, antigen presentation, and inflammation [83–85]. In mammals, cystatin C is involved in the defense against pathogen [86]. Currently, cystatin sequence has been found in ticks, from cDNA library obtained from salivary glands of *Ixodes scapularis* [82, 87–90]. The cystatin (sialostatin L) obtained from *I. scapularis* cDNA library was reported in tick saliva affected by proteolytic activity in infestation sites [88]. Moreover, SI-alostatin L, during tick blood feeding, has an important role as anti-inflammatory and in the inhibition of cytotoxic T-cell proliferation, contributing to feeding and pathogen transmission. On the other hand, cystatin RNAi-mediated silencing assay demonstrated that *Amblyomma americanum* reduced the ability to feed and evade the host immune response [87]. Recently, cystatins were shown to be expressed in ticks' salivary glands and other tissues, where they play an important role in the immune response [89, 90]. Moreover, in hard tick *R. microplus*, cystatin genes show expression in the fat body and ovary and protein expression in salivary glands, fat body, and ovary [89]. However, a possible role of the cystatin in several tissues in ticks still remains unknown. In this regard, novel cystatins from midgut were described in *Haemaphysalis longicornis* that show inhibitory activity against cysteine proteases [90]. In this regard, some assays demonstrate that *Babesis gibsoni* LPS injection is capable to increase the expression in the midgut in adult and larval ticks.

5. Nitric oxide and oxidative stress

5.1. Nitric oxide synthase

The nitric oxide (NO) is an unstable radical, capable to act with a key factor in several physiological and pathological pathways, and it is synthesized by the nitric oxide synthase (NOS) [91]. In invertebrates, including ticks, NO is related with a cytotoxic action against pathogens from hemocytes, derivates to phagocyte process during microbial infection [92]. Now, three NOS isoforms have been described: the classic isoform inducible nitric oxide synthase (iNOS), the endothelial isoform (eNOS), and the neuronal isoform (nNOS) [91, 93]. Currently, the gene that codified for NOS has been identified and cloned from the insects: *Drosophila melanogaster, Anopheles stephensi, Anopheles gambiae*, and *Rhodnius prolixus*, suggesting the NO activity is present in these arthropods [94–98]. Moreover, the activity of NOS was reported in the salivary gland of hematophagous insect *Rhodnius prolixus*, and the enzyme activity was FAD, NADPH, tetrahydrobiopterin, calmodulin, and Ca^{2+} dependent, suggesting high functionality, similar to NOS enzyme expressed in vertebrates [99]. Likewise, *Litopenaeus vannamei* shrimp is capable of producing nitric oxide, in response to *Vibrio harveyi* inoculation, derivates to NOS activity [93]. In ticks, the activity of eNOS enzyme was reported in *Dermacentor variabilis* salivary glands, and by *in silico* analysis, the presence of NOS gene sequence was demonstrated in *Ixodes scapularis* embryonated eggs [91, 100].

5.2. Oxidative stress and detoxifying protein

In hematophagous arthropods, blood ingestion is the determinant of survival. However, during feeding and digestion, several toxic molecules are produced, such as reactive nitrogen species (RNOS) and reactive oxygen species (ROS) [101]. The protection against nitrosative and oxidative stress is carried out by detoxification agents, produced largely by the midgut epithelial cells. In many insects, enzymes such as peroxiredoxins, catalases, and many members of antioxidant peroxidase family function as antioxidant agents. However, in arthropods, as in many organisms, the microbial infections are capable to induce oxidative stress. Suppression of pathogen ROS and RNOS induction in midgut facilitates the infection and microbial tissue dispersion [102]. Interestingly, many arthropods have the capacity of enhancing ROS and RNOS against pathogen infection while simultaneously protecting their tissue cells with antioxidants. In this regard, the oxidize enzyme nicotinamide adenide dinucleotide phosphate (NADPH) of *D. melanogaster*, known as dual oxidase (dDuox), is capable to kill and/or inhibit the pathogen proliferation, through the oxidative burst [103]. Moreover, the glutathione S-transferases (GST) family plays an important role during oxidative stress caused by pathogens, through detoxification enzyme reactions and, in turn, removing the formatted ROS and RNOS [104]. In midgut from *D. variabilis* tick, GST isoforms DvGST1 and DvGST2 are upregulated during blood ingestion [105], and during the *B. burgdorferi* infection in tick *I. ricinus*, several GTSs are overexpressed in response to bacterial invasion [106]. In ticks, other detoxification enzymes have been reported, such as glutaredoxins, glutathione peroxidases, phospholipid-hydroperoxidases, thioredoxins, and one superoxide dismutase [107–109]. However, in ticks, the precise role in antimicrobial control of detoxification agents is still unclear.

5.3. Phenol oxidase and melanization

In arthropods, mechanical injury or the presence of foreign objects including pathogens results in melanin deposition around the damaged tissue or around the foreign object that in turn forms a capsule isolating the foreign particle. Melanins are molecules produced in the hemolymph by different types of hemocytes. The key enzyme for the melanization process is the phenol oxidase (PO). The metabolic pathway is initiated by hydroxylation of phenylalanine to tyrosine, followed by a series of reactions, resulting in 5,6-indolquinones, synthesized to phenol quinones, and these quinones polymerize to form melanin. The production of melanin is noticed by a dark and/or blackened color in the arthropod [110–112]. The signaling pathway starts with a hemocyte prophenol oxidase enzyme (PPO) synthesis (PO inactive form) that results in the conversion of the PPO into the active form by serine protease cascade [113]. This molecular system is capable to recognize picomolar of bacterial lipopolysaccharide (LPS), peptide glycans, and fungi β-1,3-glucane. The intermediary components of this pathway, such as semiquinones, ROS, and melanin, are all very toxic to pathogens [114]. On the other hand, the PPO-PO pathway in tick is little known. However, at the present, some studies in *Amblyomma americanum, Dermacentor variabilis*, and *Ixodes scapularis* ticks report the presence of genes involved in the PPO-PO pathway; however, the enzymatic activity has not been reported [29]. In the tick *O. moubata*, the PO enzyme has been reported in hemolymph plasma and in the fourth of ecdysiast nymphs [28]. However, currently, the presence of PO in ticks is controversial.

6. Molecular approaches to tick immunology

6.1. Regulation of innate immune system in ticks

The innate immune systems represent one aspect in a generalized response to several pathogens and are composed of individual factors. This variability has a particular behavior in each tick. The principal components are the hemolymph and hemocytes; however, they are not the only factors. The response depends on the pathogen type, tissue, sex, life cycle phases, and tick species, among others. In this regard, innate immunity starts when membrane receptors recognize component characteristics of bacterial cell surfaces as peptidoglycans or lipoteichoic acid, which leads to synthesis of antimicrobial peptides (AMPs) as defensins, cecropins, attacins, and lysozyme that disrupt the cell wall structure, leading to cell death [2]. Other components in the fungi cell wall are beta-1-3-glucans and beta-1-3 mannose or 2-keto-3-deoxyoctonate LPS, characteristic of Gram-negative bacteria, leading to soluble lectin synthesis [2]. These cell wall components and foreign molecular structures are known as pathogen-associated molecular patterns (PAMPs) [2, 115]. In *D. variabilis* tick, different analyses show 56 genes involved in the immune response; however, these genes do not appear to be regulated. In sexual term, transcriptome analysis in the male reproductive structures of this tick showed seven contigs related to a dual reproductive and immune response [116]. However, the complete role of these peptides is still unknown, but their presence in seminal fluids suggests a role in the clearing of bacteria introduced during mating [117]. In the tissues, the immune response includes several factors such as AMPs, peritrophic membrane, proteases, and protease inhibitors, lectins, detoxificant proteins, and oxidative stress [3]. Transcriptome analyses in *D. variabilis* midgut show 8 transcripts related to the innate immune response, of which one protein (MD-2) is involved in lipid-domain recognition, lectins, and in turn involved in inhibition of macrophage activation [118]. Moreover, transcriptome analyses of tick salivary glands found AMPs, proteases, and protease inhibitors related to innate immune response [119–121]. The synganglion transcriptome of *D. variabilis* contains 0.27–1.15% peptides, depending on the gene ontology, that represent between 4 and 11 genes [122] and includes AMPs, proteases, lectins, protease inhibitors, and regulatory Toll-like proteins [116]. On the other hand, the widespread response has been initiated by hemocyte cell pathogen recognition carried out by the presence of microbe-associated microbial patterns (MAMPs), expressed in pathogen's membrane surface. However, in ticks, the hemocyte receptors to MAMP's recognition are still unknown, but analyses reveal similar receptors to those identified in insects [26]. In this regard, homologs to peptidoglycan receptor proteins (PGRPs), Gram-negative–binding proteins (GNBPs), and gal-lectins have been reported [123]. To identify the pathogen type, the hemocyte cells need to be activated, using specific receptors that result in a specific signaling pathway [116]. The fruit fly *D. melanogaster* has been used as a genetic model to elucidate the activation of the innate immune system, which is an evolutionarily conserved mechanism in eukaryotes. Drosophila has three pathways involved in an immune response: Toll, Imd, and Hop, homologs to TLR, TNFα, and Jak/STAT in mammals [124]. Different components of these three signaling pathways were found in tick's database, such as in Toll pathway, Toll, MyD88 and Pelle. In *Drosophila* model, the fungal pathogens and Gram-positive bacteria activate the Toll cascade, which is composed of different Toll-like receptors (TLRs) capable of recognizing diverse types of PAMPs [2, 115, 125, 126]. After pathogen recognition, intermediate effectors such as myeloid differentiation factor 88 (MyDD88), Tube, and Pelle are activated followed by activation of transcription factor Dorsal (homolog of NF-kB) and Dorsal-related immunity factor (Dif) that translocates into the nucleus and regulates the AMP synthesis [126]. From the Imd pathway, Dredd, Caspar, and Relish have been found. Gram-negative bacteria infection activates the Imd cascade through the recognition of DAP-type peptidoglycan in the membrane protein peptidoglycan (PGRP-LE) [115, 125] and activates molecules such as TAB2/TAK1, JNK, IKK, and Relish inducing the transcription of AMP [115, 126]. Finally, from the Hop pathway, JAK and STAT have been found [123]. In the absence of infection, a selective repression of this IMD/Toll-dependent AMP pathways is achieved by the home box gene Caudal [127, 128]. Recently, the RNA interference (RNAi) pathway has been described that regulates the immune system in arthropods including ticks. This process is crucial in the innate response to viruses that infect and are transmitted by ticks [129]. In *Drosophila*, the RNAi mechanism is related to a virus penetration and regulation of innate immune response in the midgut. The RNAi pathway in ticks is unknown; however, its components are described in some ticks [130], as RNAi has been used to silence genes involved in several mechanisms, suggesting that RNAi pathway is active in some tick species, which would explain the different capacity of ticks to transfer several viruses [129].

6.2. Advance in molecular, functional genomics and proteomics in tick-host-pathogen interaction

Advances in gene identification and expression in tick tissues are being achieved by the use of expressed sequence tag (EST). The EST analyses correspond to partial sequence of acid nucleic from different random clones included in a cDNA library, obtained from the interest tissue mRNA [131]. The analyses include the translation of EST sequence to amino acid sequence and compared with a public genome database. Interestingly, salivary gland genes of ticks show differential expression during blood ingestion, suggesting that processes are involved in homeostasis, tissue remodeling, immune defenses, angiogenesis, and the facilitation of the transmissible pathogen establishment [132]. The EST library from unfed hard tick larvae of *R. microplus* was the first study reported [133]. However, 234 unique ESTs were identified, and 39% of them were not found in genome database. In *A. americanum*, cDNA libraries showed that 1462 and 480 ESTs (adult and larvae respectively) presented 56% to no-similarity identified in encoded proteins [134]. On the other hand, *R. microplus* gene expression analyses from cDNA library obtained from RNA tissue larvae exposed to different stimuli and infected with *Babesia* showed that 8270 unique sequences were identified to 11,520 total sequenced clones and presented a 44% of shared similarity to database sequences [135]. A meta-analysis was done, which describes the transcripts from salivary glands of several species of ticks, including the salivary gland transcripts from unfed male of *I. ricinus* and *A. americanus*; fed female of *I. pacificus* and *A. variegatum*; unfed female and unfed-fed nymphs of *I. scapularis*; and finally unfed males and fed female of *Dermacentor andersoni*. All tick groups analyzed were from different ages and different feeding times, or unfed. The results showed that the secreted proteins comprised 49% from which 15% were no match with any gene reported *in silico* analyses. Interestingly, transposable elements were found in 0.5% of the transcripts, which suggest gene rearrangements. In the exclusive case of females, differential gene expressions of transcripts were showed. The unfed female showed no change in expression, while fed female showed the highest number of overexpressed variants. All biologically relevant genes are likely redundant and encode antigenic variants, in turn identifying gene families involved in hemostatic deregulation. Other identified genes include cystatins, lectins, cysteine and glycine-rich peptides, and protease inhibitors [119, 132, 136–138]. A very important finding in *R. appendiculatus* tick showed that tick-borne pathogen presence did not modify the gene expression. In this regard, no significant differences were found in the expressed transcripts of 9162 ESTs from salivary glands of *R. appendiculatus* uninfected, compared with the 9844 ESTs obtained from salivary gland of *R. appendiculatus* infected with *Theileria parva* [139]. Currently, the genome sequence of several arthropod vectors including ticks is under development, and partial results of *I. scapularis* sequencing efforts reveal that deer tick genome is approximately 2.1 Gbp; likewise, the hard tick *R. microplus* genome contains 7.1 Gbp [140]. It is remarkable that cattle tick genome is more than twice the size of the human genome that contains 3–2 Gbp [141]; furthermore, the cattle tick genomes are larger than most insect species genomes.

7. Future directions

The ever-increasing knowledge of the immune system biology of vertebrates represents an important foundation in the research and development of advanced vaccines, new drugs, as well as the search for new targets for chemical or drug treatments of infectious diseases, which have contributed to the control of several human and livestock pathogens. Unfortunately, the immune system of invertebrates, especially, arthropod vectors like ticks, and their relationship with their pathogens, and infectious diseases they transmit, have been little explored. In this regard, the knowledge of mechanisms, molecules, and cells, as well as the regulation of immune response signaling pathways, represents an advance in designing control strategies that will contribute to improve livestock production and animal health. Currently, studies in insects and the molecular tool development help us to advance in the research to arthropod immune system regulation; however, there are many knowledge gaps about the ticks' immune response. Elucidation of the different molecular pathways and their regulation in ticks' immunobiology brings us closer to understand the role in the transmission of various infectious agents. Now, all transcriptome analyses and whole-genome sequencing represent powerful methodologies for understanding the biology, evolutionary relationships, and host-vector-pathogen interaction. The use of DNA/RNA sequencing modern tools could potentiate the discovery of different aspects that remain unsolved in tick biology, for the elucidation of the paradigms that currently remain unknown.

Acknowledgements

Hugo Aguilar-Díaz acknowledges the support given by Programa de Retenciones, Consejo Nacional de Ciencia y Tecnología (CONACYT), No. MOD- ORD-27 PCI-187-11-15.

Author details

Hugo Aguilar-Díaz* and Raquel Cossío-Bayúgar

*Address all correspondence to: hugoaguilar@ciencias.unam.mx

Instituto Nacional de Investigaciones Forestales, Agrícolas y Pecuarias, Centro Nacional de Investigación Disciplinaria en Parasitología Veterinaria Carretera Federal Cuernavaca-Cuautla, Jiutepec, Morelos, México

References

[1] Sonenshine DE, Roe RM. Biology of Ticks. 2nd ed. Vol. 2. New York: Oxford University Press; 2013. 496 pp. ISBN 978-0-19-974406-0 (hard cover)

[2] Hynes WL. How ticks control microbes. Innate immune response. In: Sonenshine DE, Roe RM, editors. Biology of Ticks. 2nd ed. Vol. 2. New York: Oxford University Press; 2014. p. 129-146. ISBN: 978-0-19-974406-0

[3] Sonenshine DE, Hynes WL. Molecular characterization and related aspects of the innate immune response in ticks. Frontiers in Bioscience. 2008;**1**(13):7046-7063

[4] DeMar T. Innate immunity in ticks: A review. Journal of Acarological Society of Japan. 2006;**15**(2):109-127

[5] Johns R, Sonenshine DE, Hynes WL. Control of bacterial infections in the hard tick Dermacentor variabilis (Acari: Ixodidae): Evidence for the existence of antimicrobial proteins in tick hemolymph. Journal of Medical Entomology. 1998;**35**:458-464

[6] Johns R, Sonenshine DE, Hynes WL. Response of the tick Dermacentor variabilis (Acari: Ixodidae) to hemocoelic inoculation of *Borrelia burgdorferi* (Spirochetales). Journal of Medical Entomology. 2000;**37**:265-270

[7] Johns R. Tick Immunology and its Influence on Vector Competence [PhD Dissertation]. Norfolk, VA, USA: Department of Biological Sciences, Old Dominion University; 2003

[8] Inoue N, Hanada K, Tsuji N, Igarashi I, Nagasawa H, Mikami T, Fujisaki K. Characterization ofphagocytic hemocytes in Ornithodoros moubata (Acari: Ixodidae). Journal of Medical Entomology. 2001;**38**:514-519

[9] Borovickova B, Hypša V. Ontogeny of tick hemocytes: A comparative analysis of Ixodes ricinus and Ornithodoros moubata. Experimental & Applied Acarology. 2005;**35**: 317-333

[10] Gillespie JP, Kanost MR, Trenczek T. Biological mediators of insect immunity. Annual Review of Entomology. 1997;**42**:611-643

[11] Kuhn KH, Haug T. Ultrastructural, cytochemical, and immunocytochemical characterization of haemocytes of the hard tick Ixodes ricinus (Acari: Chelicerata). Cell and Tissue Research. 1994;**277**:493-504

[12] Brinton LP, Burgdorfer W. Fine structure of normal hemocytes in Dermacentor andersoni stiles (Acari: Ixodidae). Journal of Parasitology. 1971;**57**:1110-1127

[13] Sonenshine DE. Biology of Ticks. Vol. 2. Oxford: Oxford University Press; 1993. 465 pp

[14] Zhioua E, Lebrun RA, Johnson PW, Ginsberg HS. Ultrastructure of the hemocytes of Iodes scapularis (Acari: Ixodidae). Acarologia. 1996;**37**:173-179

[15] Borovičkova B, Hypša V. Ontogeny of tick hemocytes: A comparative analysis of Ixodes ricinus and Ornithodoros moubata. Experimental and Applied Acarology. 2005;**35**:317-333

[16] Lamprou I, Mamali I, Dallas K, Fertakis V, Lampropoulou M, Marmaras VJ. Distinct signaling pathways promote phagocytosis of bacteria, latex beads and lipopolysaccharide in medfly haemocytes. Immunology. 2007;**121**(3):314-327

[17] Pereira LS, Oliveira PL, Barja-fidalgo C, Daffre S. Production of reactive oxygen species byhemocytes from the cattle tick Boophilus microplus. Experimental Parasitology. 2001;**99**:66-72

[18] Grubhoffer L, Kovař V. Arthropod lectins: Affinity approaches in the analysis and preparation of carbohydrate binding proteins. In: Wiesner A, Dunphy GG, Marmaras VJ, Orishima I, Sugumaran M, Yamakawa M, editors. Techniques in Insect Immunology FITC-5. Fair Haven, New Jersey: SOS Publications; 1998. pp. 47-57

[19] Kovař V, Kopaček P, Grubhoffer L. Isolation and characterization of Dorin M, a lectin from plasma of the soft tick Ornithodoros moubata. Insect Biochemistry and Molecular Biology. 2000;**30**:195-205

[20] Rego ROM, Hajdušek O, Kovař V, Kopaček P, Grubhoffer L, Hypša V. Molecular cloning and comparative analysis of fibrinogen-related proteins from the soft tick Ornithodoros moubata and the hard tick Ixodes ricinus. Insect Biochemistry and Molecular Biology. 2005;**35**:991-1004

[21] Huang X, Tsuji N, Miyoshi T, Nakamura-Tsuruta S, Hirabayashi J, Fujisaki K. Molecular characterization and oligosaccharide-binding properties of a galectin from the argasid tick Ornithodoros moubata. Glycobiology. 2007;**17**:313-323

[22] Kopacek P, Hajdusek O, Buresova V. Tick as a model for the study of a primitive complement system. In: Recent Advances on Model Hosts. New York: Springer; 2012. pp. 83-93

[23] Rego RO, Hajdusek O, Kovar V, Kopacek P, Grubhoffer L, Hypsa V. Hypsa: Molecular cloning and comparative analysis of fibrinogen-related proteins from the soft tick Ornithodoros moubata and the hard tick Ixodes ricinus. Insect Biochemistry and Molecular Biology. 2005;**35**:991-1004

[24] Gandhe AS, John SH, Nagaraju J. Noduler, a novel immune up-regulated protein mediates nodulation response in insects. Journal of Immunology. 2007;**179**:6943-6951

[25] Ceraul SM, Sonenshine DE, Hynes WL. Resistance of the tick Dermacentor variabilis (Acari: Ixodidae) following challenge with the bacterium Escherichia coli (Enterobacteriales: Enterobacteriaceae). Journal of Medical Entomology. 2002;**39**:376-378

[26] Marmaras VJ, Lampropoulou M. Regulator and signaling in insect haemocyte immunity. Cellular Signalling. 2009;**21**:186-195

[27] Royet J, Meister M, Ferrandon D. Humoral and cellular responses in drosophila innate immunity. In: Ezekowitz RAB, Hoffmann JA, editors. Innate Immunity. Totowa: Humana Press Inc; 2003

[28] Kadota K, Satoh E, Ochiai M, Inoue N, Tsuji N, Igarashi I, Nagasawa H, Mikami T, Claveria FG, Fujisaki K. Existence of phenol oxidase in the argasid tick Ornithodoros moubata. Parasitology Research. 2002;**88**:781-784

[29] Zhioua E, Yeh MT, LeBrun RA. Assay for pheonloxidase activity in Amblyomma americanum, Dermacentor variabilis, and Ixodes scapularis. Journal of Parasitology. 1997;**83**:553-554

[30] Eggenberger LR, Lamoreaux WJ, Coons LB. Hemocytic encapsulation of implants in the tick Dermacentor variabilis. Experimental and Applied Acarology. 1990;**9**:279-287

[31] Stanley D. Prostaglandins and other eicosanoids in insects: Biological significance. Annual Review of Entomology. 2006;**51**:25-44

[32] Kopacek P, Hajdusek O, Buresova V, Daffre S. Tick innate immunity. In: Soderhall K, editor. Invertebrate Immunity. Austin, TX: Landes Bioscience and Springer; 2010. pp. 137-162

[33] Gudderra NP, Sonenshine DE, Apperson CS, Roe RM. Hemolymph proteins in ticks. Journal of Insect Physiology. 2002;**48**:269-278

[34] Vierstraete E, Cerstiaens A, Baggerman G, Van den Bergh G, De Loof A, Schoofs L. Proteomics in Drosophila melanogaster: First 2D database of larval hemolymph proteins. Biochemical and Biophysical Research Communications. 2003;**304**:831-838

[35] Fogaca AC, Lorenzini DM, Kaku LM, Esteves E, Bulet P, Daffre S. Cysteine-rich antimicrobialpeptides of three cattle tick Boophilus microplus: Isolation, structural characterization and tissue expression profile. Developmental and Comparative Immunology. 2004;**28**:191-200

[36] Lai R, Takeuchi H, Lomas LO, Jonczy J, Rigden DJ, Rees HH, Turner PC. A new type of antimicrobialprotein with multiple histidines from the hard tick, Amblyomma hebraeum. FASEB Journal. 2004b;**18**:1447-1449

[37] Fogaca AC, Almeida IC, Eberlin MN, Tanaka AS, Bulet P, Daffre S. Ixodidin, a novel antimicrobialpeptide from the hemocytes of the cattle tick Boophilus microplus with inhibitory activity against serine proteinases. Peptides. 2006;**27**:667-674

[38] Pichu S, Ribeiro JMC, Mather TN. Purification and characterization of a novel salivary antimicrobial peptide from the tick, Ixodes scapularis. Biochemical and Biophysical Research Communications. 2009;**390**:511-515

[39] Lai R, Lomas LO, Jonczy J, Turner PC, Rees HH. Two novel non-cationic defensin-like antimicrobial peptides from hemolymph of the female tick, Amblyomma hebraeum. Biochemistry Journal. 2004a;**379**:681-685

[40] Ganz T. Defensins: Antimicrobial peptides of innate immunity. Nature Reviews. Immunology. 2003;**3**:710-720

[41] Johns R, Sonenshine DE, Hynes WL. Identification of a defensin from the hemolymph of the American dog tick, Dermacentor variabilis. Insect Biochemistry and Molecular Biology. 2001;**31**:857-865

[42] Nakajima Y, Van der Goes van Naters-Yasui A, Taylor D, Yamakawa M. Two isoforms of a member of the arthropod defensin family from the soft tick, Ornithodoros moubata (Acari: Argasidae). Insect Biochemistry and Molecular Biology. 2001;**31**:747-751

[43] Cociancich S, Ghazi A, Hetru C, Hoffmann JA, Letellier L. Insect defensin, an inducible antibacterial peptide, forms voltage-dependent channels in Micrococcus luteus. The Journal of Biological Chemistry. 1993;**268**:19239-19245

[44] Hynes WL, Ceraul SM, Todd SM, Sonenshine DE. A defensing-like gene expressed in the black-legged tick, Ixodes scapularis. Medical and Veterinary Entomology. 2005;**19**:339-344

[45] Nakajima Y, Saido-Sakanaka H, Taylor D, Yamakawa M. Up-regulated humoral immune response in the soft tick, Ornithodoros moubata (Acari: Argasidae). Parasitology Research. 2003;**91**:476-481

[46] Nakajima Y, Taylor D, Yamakawa M. Involvement of antibacterial peptide defensin in tick midgut defense. Experimental & Applied Acarology. 2002;**28**:135-140

[47] Simser JA, Macaluso KR, Mulenga A, Azad AF. Immune-responsive lysozymes from hemocytes of the American dog tick, Dermacentor variabilis and an embryonic cell line of the Rocky Mountain wood tick, D. andersoni. Insect Biochemistry and Molecular Biology. 2004;**34**:1235-1246

[48] Sonenshine DE, Hynes WL, Ceraul SM, Mitchell R, Benzine T. Host blood proteins and peptides in the midgut of the tick Dermacentor variabilis contribute to bacterial control. Experimental & Applied Acarology. 2005;**36**:207-223

[49] Ceraul SM, Dreher-Lesnick SM, Gillespie JJ, Rahman MS, Azad AF. New tick defensin isoform and antimicrobial gene expression in response to Rickettsia montanensis challenge. Infection and Immunity. 2007;**75**:1973-1983

[50] Tanaka T, Kawano S, Nakao S, Umemiya-Shirafuji R, Rahman MM, Boldbaatar D, Battur B, Liao M, Fujisaki K. The identification and characterization of lysozyme from the hard tick Haemaphysalis longicornis. Ticks and Tick-borne Diseases. 2010;**1**:178-185

[51] Grunclova L, Fouquier H, Hypsa V, Kopacek P. Lysozyme from the gut of the soft tick Ornithodoros moubata: The sequence, phylogeny and post-feeding regulation. Developmental and Comparative Immunology. 2003;**27**:651-660

[52] Kopaček P, Vogt R, Jindrak L, Weise C, Safarik I. Purification and characterization of the lysozyme from the gut of the soft tick Ornithodoros moubata. Insect Biochemistry and Molecular Biology. 1999;**29**:989-997

[53] Yu D, Sheng Z, Xu X, Li J, Yang H, Liu Z, Rees HH, Lai R. A novel antimicrobial peptide from salivary glands of the hard tick, Ixodes sinensis. Peptides. 2005;**27**:31-35

[54] Grubhoffer L, Kovar V, Rudenko N. Tick lectins: Structural and functional properties. Parasitology (Suppl). 2004;**129**:S113-S125

[55] Chen SC, Yen CH, Yeh MMS, Huang CH, Liu TY. Biochemical properties and cDNA cloning of two new lectins from the plasma of Tachypleus tridentatus. Journal of Biological Chemistry. 2001;**276**:9631-9639

[56] Natori S. Insect lectins and innate immunity. Advances in Experimental Medicine and Biology. 2001;**484**:223-228

[57] Rego RO, Kovar V, Kopacek P, Weise C, Man P, Sauman I, Grubhoffer L. The tick plasma lectin, Dorin M, is a fibrinogen-related molecule. Insect Biochemistry and Molecular Biology. 2006;**36**:291-299

[58] Munderloh U, Jauron SD, Kurtti TJ. The tick: A different kind of host for human pathogens. In: Goodman JL, Dennis DT, Sonenshine DE, editors. Tick-Borne Diseases of Humans. Washington, D.C: ASM Press; 2005

[59] Vasta GR, Marchalonis JJ. Humoral recognition factors in the arthropoda. The specificity of chelicerate serum lectins. American Zoology. 1983;**23**:157-171

[60] Vereš J, Grubhoffer L. Detection and partial characterization of a new plasma lectin in the hemolymph of the tick Ornithodoros tartakovskyi. Microbios Letters. 1990;**45**:61-64

[61] Grubhoffer L, Veres J, Dusbabek F. Lectins as the molecular factors of recognition and defense reactions of ticks. In: Dusbabek F, Bukva V, editors. Modern Acarology. Vol. 2. The Hague: Praque and SPB Academic Publishing; 1991. pp. 381-388

[62] Grubhoffer L, Kovař V. Arthropod lectins: Affinity approaches in the analysis and preparation of carbohydrate binding proteins. In: Wiesner A, Dunphy GG, Marmaras VJ, Morishima I, Sugumaran M, Yamakawa M, editors. Techniques in Insect Immunology FITC-5. Fair Haven, New Jersey: SOS Publications; 1998. pp. 47-57

[63] Kamwendo SP, Ingram GA, Musisi FL, Molyneux DH. Haemagglutinin activity in tick (Rhipicephalus appendiculatus) haemolymph and extracts of gut and salivary glands. Annals of Tropical Medicine and Parasitology. 1993;**87**:303-305

[64] Kamwendo SP, Musis FL, Trees AJ, Molyneux DH. Effect of haemagglutinin (lectin) inhibitory sugars in Theileria parva infection in Rhipicephalus appendiculatus. International Journal for Parasitology. 1995;**25**:29-35

[65] Uhliř J, Grubhoffer L, Volf P. Novel agglutinin in the midgut of the tick Ixodes ricinus. Folia Parasitologica. 1996;**43**:233-239

[66] Miyoshi T, Tsuji N, Islam MK, Huang X, Motobu M, Alim MA, Fujisaki K. Molecular and reverse genetic characterization of serine proteinase induced hemolysis in the midgut of the ixodid tick Haemaphysalis longicornis. Journal of Insect Physiology. 2007;**53**:195-203

[67] Mulenga A, Misao O, Sugimoto C. Three serine proteinases from midguts of the hard tick Rhipicephalus appendiculatus; cDNA cloning and preliminary characterization. Experimental & Applied Acarology. 2003;**29**:151-164

[68] Boldbaatar D, Sikasunge C, Battsetseg B, Xuanand X, Fujisaki K. Molecular cloning and functional characterization of an aspartic protease from the hard tick Haemaphysalis longicornis. Insect Biochemistry and Molecular Biology. 2006;**36**:25-36

[69] Willot E, Tran HQ. Zinc and Manduca sexta hemocyte functions. Journal of Insect Science. 2002;**2**:1-9

[70] JF. Anderson, DE. Sonenshine, J. Valenzuela, Exploring the mialome of ticks: An annotated catalogue of midgut transcripts from the hard tick Dermacentor variabilis (Acari: Ixodidae). 2008. Submitted

[71] Simser JA, Mulenga A, Macaluso KR, Azad AF. An inmune responsive factor D-like serine protein as a homologue identified from the American dog tick, Dermacentor variabilis. Insect Molecular Biology. 2004b;**13**:25-35

[72] Jiang H, Kanost MR. The clip-domain family of serine proteinases in arthropods. Insect Biochemistry and Molecular Biology. 2000;**30**:95-105

[73] Xu WY, Huang FS, Hao HX, Duan JH, Qiu ZW. Two serine proteases from Anopheles dirus haemocytes exhibit changes in transcript abundance after infection of an incompatible rodent malaria parasite, Plasmodium yoelii. Veterinary Parasitology. 2006;**139**:93-101

[74] Kawabata S, Tokunaga F, Kugi Y, Motoyama S, Miura Y, Hirata M, Iwanaga S. Limulus factor D, a43-kDa protein isolated from horseshoe crab hemocytes, is a serine protease homologue with antimicrobial activity. FEBS Letters. 1996;**398**:146-150

[75] Armstrong PB. The contribution of proteinase inhibitors to immune defense. Trends in Immunology. 2001;**22**:47-52

[76] Kanost MR, Jiang H. Protease inhibitors in invertebrate immunity. In: Soderhall K, Iwanaga S, Vanta G, editors. New Directions in Invertebrate Immunology. Fair Haven, NJ: SOS Publications; 1996. pp. 155-173

[77] Mulenga A, Khumthong R, Blandon MA. Molecular and expression analysis of a family of the *Amblyomma americanum* tick *Lospins*. The Journal of Experimental Biology. 2007; **210**(18):3188-3198

[78] Polanowski A, Wilusz T. Serine proteinase inhibitors from insect hemolymph. Acta Biochimica Polonica. 1996;**43**:445-453

[79] Milenga A, Sugimoto C, Onuma M. Issue in tick vaccine development: Identification an characterization of potential candidate vaccine antigens. Microbes and Infection. 2000;**2**:1353-1361

[80] Armstrong PB, Quigley JP. Alpha2-macroglobulin: An evolutionarily conserved arm of theinnate immune system. Developmental and Comparative Immunology. 1999;**23**: 375-390

[81] Saravanan T, Weise C, Sojka D, Kopáček P. Molecular cloning, structure and bait region splice variants of alpha 2-macroglobulin from the soft tick Ornithodoros moubata. Insect Biochemistry and Molecular Biology. 2003;**33**:841-851

[82] Valenzuela JG, Francischetti IM, Pham VM, Garfield MK, Mather TN, Ribeiro JM. Exploring the sialome of the tick Ixodes scapularis. Journal of Experimental Biology. 2002;**205**:2843-2864

[83] Honey K, Rudensky AY. Lysosomal cysteine proteases regulate antigen presentation. Nature Reviews. Immunology. 2003;**3**:472-482

[84] Lombardi G, Burzyn D, Mundinano J, Berguer P, Bekinschtein P, Costa H, Castillo LF, Goldman A, Meiss R, Reinheckel I, Hagemann TS, Dollwet-Mack S, Martinez E, Lohmuller T, Zlatkovic G, Tobin DJ, Maas-Szabowski N, Peters C. The lysosomal cysteine protease cathepsin L regulates keratinocyte proliferation by control of growth factor recycling. Journal of Cell Science. 2005;**118**:3387-3395

[85] Reddy VY, Zhang QY, Weiss SJ. Pericellular mobilization of the tissue-destructive cysteine proteinases, cathepsins B, L, and S, by human monocyte-derived macrophages. Proceedings of the National Academy of Sciences of the United States of America. 1995;**92**:3849-3853

[86] Olsson SL, Ek B, Bjork I. The affinity and kinetics of inhibition of cysteine proteinases by intact recombinant bovine cystatin C. Biochimica et Biophysica Acta. 1999;**1432**:73-81

[87] Karim S, Miller NJ, Valenzuela J, Sauer JR, Mather TN. RNAi-mediated gene silencing to assess the role of synaptobrevin and cystatin in tick blood feeding. Biochemical and Biophysical Research Communications. 2005;**334**:1336-1342

[88] Kotsyfakis M, Sa-Nunes A, Francischetti IMB, Mather TN, Andersen JF, Ribeiro JMC. Antiinflammatory and immunosuppressive activity of sialostatin L, a salivary cystatin from the tick Ixodes scapularis. Journal of Biological Chemistry. 2006;**281**:26298-26307

[89] Lima CA, Sasaki SD, Tanaka AS. Bmcystatin, a cysteine proteinase inhibitor characterized from the tick Boophilus microplus. Biochemical and Biophysical Research Communications. 2006;**347**:44-50

[90] Zhou J, Ueda M, Umemiya R, Battsetseg B, Boldbaatar D, Xuan X, Fujisaki K. A secreted cystatin fromthe tick Haemaphysalis longicornis and its distinct expression patterns in relation to innate immunity. Insect Biochemistry and Molecular Biology. 2006;**36**:527-535

[91] Gonzalez-Domenech CM, Munoz-Chapuli R. Molecular evolution of nitric oxide synthases in metazoans. Comparative Biochemistry and Physiology. Part D. Genomics & Proteomics, Amsterdam-NL. 2010;**5**(4):295-301

[92] Faraldo AC et al. Nitric oxide production in blowfly hemolymph after yeast inoculation. Nitric Oxide. 2005;**13**:240-246

[93] Chen T et al. Nitric oxide as an antimicrobial molecule against Vibrio harveyi infection in the hepatopancreas of Pacific white shrimp, Litopenaeus vannamei. Fish & Shellfish Immunology. 2015;**42**:114-120

[94] Regulski M, Tully T. Molecular and biochemical characterization of dNOS: A drosophila Ca^{2+}/calmodulin-dependent nitric oxide synthase. Proceedings of the National Academy of Sciences of the United States of America. 1995;**92**:90722-90726

[95] Yuda M et al. cDNA cloning, expression and characterization of nitric oxide synthase from the salivary glands of the blood-sucking insect Rhodnius prolixus. European Journal of Biochemistry. 1996;**242**:807-812

[96] Luckhart S et al. The mosquito Anopheles stephensi limits malaria parasite development with inducible synthesis of nitric oxide. Proceedings of the National Academy of Sciences of the United States of America. 1998;**95**:5700-5705

[97] Luckhart S, Rosenberg R. Gene structure and polymorphism of an invertebrate nitric oxide synthase gene. Gene. 1999;**232**:25-34

[98] Imamura M, Yang J, Yamakawa M. cDNA cloning, characterization and gene expression of nitric oxide synthase from the silkworm, Bombyx mori. Insect Biochemistry and Molecular Biology. 2002;**11**:257-265

[99] Ribeiro JMC, Nussenzveig RH. Nitric oxide synthase activity from a hematophagous insect salivary gland. FEBS journal, oxford. GB. 1993;**330**:165-168

[100] Bhattacharya ST, Bayakly N, Lloyd R, Benson MT, Davenport J, Fitzgerald MEC, Rothschild M, Lamoreaux WJ, Coons LB. Nitric oxide synthase and cGMP activity in the salivary glands of the American dog tick Dermacentor variabilis. Experimental Parasitology. 2000;**94**:111-120

[101] DeJong RJ, Miller LM, Molina-Cruz A, Gupta L, Kumar S, Barillas-Mury C. Reactive oxygen species detoxification by catalase is a major determinant of fecundity in the mosquito Anopheles gambiae. Proceedings of the National Academy of Sciences of the United States of America. 2007;**104**:2121-2126

[102] Peterson TM, Luckhart S. A mosquito 2-cysperoxiredoxin protects against nitrosative and oxidative stresses associated with malaria parasite infection. Free Radical Biology and Medicine. 2006;**40**:1067-1082

[103] Chalk R, Townson H, Natori S, Desmond H, Ham PJ. Purification of an insect defensin from themosquito, Aedes aegypti. Insect Biochemistry and Molecular Biology. 1994;**24**:403-410

[104] Enayti AA, Ranson H, Hemingway J. Insect glutathione transferases and insecticide resistance. Insect Molecular Biology. 2005;**14**:3-8

[105] Dreher-Lesnick SM, Mulenga A, Simser JA, Azad AF. Differential expression of two glutathione transferases identified from the American dog tick, Dermacentor variabilis. Insect Molecular Biology. 2006;**15**:445-453

[106] Rudenko N, Golovchenko M, Edwards MJ, Grubhoffer L. Differential expression of Ixodes ricinus tick genes induced by blood feeding or Borrelia burgdorferi infection. Journal of Medical Entomology. 2005;**42**:36-41

[107] Cossío-Bayúgar R, Miranda E, Holman P. Molecular cloning of a phospholipid-hydroperoxide glutathione peroxidase gene from the tick, Boophilus microplus (Acari: Ixodidae). Insect Biochemistry and Molecular Biology. 2005;**35**(12):1378-1387. DOI: 10.1016/j.ibmb.2005.08.008

[108] Cossío-Bayúgar R, Castro-Saines E, García-Vázquez Z, Miranda E. 2003.Glutathione peroxidase enzyme detection from susceptible and acaricide resistant *Boophilus microplus* ticks on sds polyacrilamide gels. V International SEMINAR IN Animal Parasitology,

Mérida, Yucatán, México; Octubre 1-3, 2003. pp. 144-149. Pero congresos no estamos reportando

[109] Anderson JF, Sonenshine DE, Valenzuela J. Exploring the mialome of ticks: An annotated catalogue of midgut transcripts from the hard tick Dermacentor variabilis (Acari: Ixodidae). 2008. Submitted

[110] Napolitano A, Di Donato P, Prota G. New regulatory mechanisms in the biosynthesis of pheomelanins: Rearrangement vs. redox exchange reaction routes of a transient 2H-1,4-benzothiazine-o-quinonimine intermediate. Biochimica et Biophysical Acta. 2000;**1475**:47-54

[111] Nappi AJ et al. Nitric oxide involvement in drosophila immunity. Nitric Oxide: Biology and Chemistry. 2000;4(4):423-430

[112] Hillyer JF, Schmidt SL, Fuchs JF, Boyle JP, Christensen BM. Age-associated mortality in immune challenged mosquitoes (Aedes aegypti) correlates with a decrease in haemocyte numbers. Cellular Microbiology. 2005;**7**:39-51

[113] Bali GK, Kaur S. Phenoloxidase activity in haemolymph of Spodoptera litura (Fabricius) mediating immune responses challenge with entomopathogenic fungus, Beauveria bassiana (Balsamo) Vuillmin. Journal of Entomology and Zoology Studies. 2013;**1**(6): 118-123

[114] Sonderhall K, Cerenius L. Role of the prophenoloxidase-activating system in invertebrate immunity. Current Opinion in Immunology. 1998;**10**:23-28

[115] Charroux B, Rival T, Narbonne/Reveau K, Royet J. Bacterial detection by Drosophila peptidoglycan recognition proteins. Microbes and Infection. 2009;**6-7**:631-636. DOI: 10.1016/j.micinf.2009.03.004

[116] Sonenshine DE, Bissinger BW, Egekwu N, Donohue KV, Khalil SM, Roe RM. First transciptome of the testis-vas deferens-male accessory gland and proteome of the spermatophore from Dermacentor variabilis (Acari: Ixodidae). PLoS One. 2011;**6**:e24711

[117] Avila FW, Sirot LK, LaFlamme BA, Rubinstein CD, Wolfner MF. Insect seminal fluid proteins: Identification and function. Annual Review of Entomology. 2011;**56**:21-40

[118] Anderson JM, Sonenchine DE, Valenzuela JG. Exploring the mialome of ticks: An annotated catalogue of midgut transcripts from the hard tick, Dermacentor variabilis (Acari: Ixodidae). BMC Genomics. 2008;**9**:552

[119] Francischetti IM, My Pham V, Mans BJ, Andersen JF, Mather TN, Lane RS, Ribeiro JM. The transcriptome of the salivary glands of the female western black-legged tick Ixodes pacificus (Acari: Ixodidae). Insect Biochemistry and Molecular Biology. 2005;**35**:1142-1161

[120] Aljamali MN, Bior AD, Sauer JR, Essenberg RC. RNA interference in ticks: A study using histamine binding protein dsRNA in the female tick Amblyomma americanum. Insect Molecular Biology. 2003;**12**:299-305

[121] Anatriello E, Riveiro JMC, De Miranda-Santos, et al. An insight into sialotranscriptome of the brown dog tick Rhipicephalus sanguineus. BMC Genomics. 2010;**11**:450

[122] Bissinger BW, Donohue KV, Khalil SMS, Grozinger CM, Sonenshine DE, Zhu J, Roe RM. Synganglion transcriptome and developmental global gene expression in adult females of the American dog tick, Dermacentor variabilis (Acari: Ixodidae). Insect Molecular Biology. 2011;**20**(4):465-491

[123] Gerardo NM, Altincicek B, Anselme C, Atamian H, Barribeau SM, De Vos M, Heddi A. Immunity and other defenses in pea aphids, Acyrthosiphon pisum. Genome Biology. 2010;**11**(2):1

[124] Pinheiro VB, Ellar DJ. How to kill a mocking bug? Cellular Microbiology. 2006;**8**(4):545-557

[125] Sonenshine DE, Roe RM. Overview: Ticks, people and animals. Biology of Ticks. 2014;**1**:3-16

[126] Valenzuela JG, Francischetti IM, Pham VM, Garfield MK, Ribeiro JM. Exploring the salivary gland transcriptome and proteome of the Anopheles stephensi mosquito. Insect Biochemistry and Molecular Biology. 2003;**33**(7):717-732

[127] Ha EM, Lee KA, Park SH, Kim SH, Nam HJ, Lee HY, Lee WJ. Regulation of DUOX by the Gαq-phospholipase Cβ-Ca^{2+} pathway in Drosophila gut immunity. Developmental Cell. 2009;**16**(3):386-397

[128] Ryu JH, Ha EM, Lee WJ. Innate immunity and gut–microbe mutualism in drosophila. Developmental & Comparative Immunology. 2010;**34**(4):369-376

[129] Karim S, Adamson SW, Simpson SJ, Casas J. RNA interference in ticks: A functional genomics tool for the study of physiology. Advances in Insect Physiology. 2012;**42**:119

[130] Kurscheid S, Lew-Tabor AE, Valle MR, Bruyeres AG, Doogan VJ, Munderloh UG, Bellgard MI. Evidence of a tick RNAi pathway by comparative genomics and reverse genetics screen of targets with known loss-of-function phenotypes in Drosophila. BMC Molecular Biology. 2009;**10**(1):1

[131] Adams MD, Kelley JM, Gocayne JD, Dubnick M, Polymeropoulos MH, Xiao H, Kerlavage AR. Complementary DNA sequencing: Expressed sequence tags and human genome project. Science. 1991;**252**(5013):1651-1656

[132] Ribeiro JM, Alarcon-Chaidez F, Francischetti IM, Mans BJ, Mather TN, Valenzuela JG, Wikel SK. An annotated catalog of salivary gland transcripts from Ixodes scapularis ticks. Insect Biochemistry and Molecular Biology. 2006;**36**(2):111-129

[133] Crampton AL, Miller C, Baxter GD, Barker SC. Expressed sequenced tags and new genes from the cattle tick, Boophilus microplus. Experimental & Applied Acarology. 1998;**22**(3):177-186

[134] Hill CA, Gutierrez JA. Analysis of the expressed genome of the lone star tick, Amblyomma americanum (Acari: Ixodidae) using an expressed sequence tag approach. Microbial & Comparative Genomics. 2000;**5**(2):89-101

[135] Guerrero FD, Miller RJ, Rousseau ME, Sunkara S, Quackenbush J, Lee Y, Nene V. BmiGI: A database of cDNAs expressed in Boophilus microplus, the tropical/southern cattle tick. Insect Biochemistry and Molecular Biology. 2005;**35**(6):585-595

[136] Bior AD, Essenberg RC, Sauer JR. Comparison of differentially expressed genes in the salivary glands of male ticks, Amblyomma americanum and Dermacentor andersoni. Insect Biochemistry and Molecular Biology. 2002;**32**(6):645-655

[137] Alarcon-Chaidez FJ, Sun J, Wikel SK. Transcriptome analysis of the salivary glands of Dermacentor andersoni stiles (Acari: Ixodidae). Insect Biochemistry and Molecular Biology. 2007;**37**(1):48-71

[138] Wikel S. Ticks and tick-borne pathogens at the cutaneous interface: Host defenses, tick countermeasures, and a suitable environment for pathogen establishment. Frontiers in Microbiology. 2013;**4**:337

[139] Nene V, Lee D, Kang'a S, Skilton R, Shah T, de Villiers E, Bishop R. Genes transcribed in the salivary glands of female Rhipicephalus appendiculatus ticks infected with Theileria parva. Insect Biochemistry and Molecular Biology. 2004;**34**(10):1117-1128

[140] Ullmann AJ, Lima CMR, Guerrero FD, Piesman J, Black WCT. Genome size and organization in the blacklegged tick, Ixodes scapularis and the southern cattle tick, Boophilus microplus. Insect Molecular Biology. 2005;**14**(2):217-222

[141] Venter JC, Adams MD, Myers EW, Li PW, Mural RJ, Sutton GG, Gocayne JD. The sequence of the human genome. Science. 2001;**291**(5507):1304-1351

Chapter 3

Genome-Based Vaccinology Applied to Bovine Anaplasmosis

Itzel Amaro-Estrada and
Sergio D. Rodríguez-Camarillo

Additional information is available at the end of the chapter

http://dx.doi.org/10.5772/intechopen.72537

Abstract

Bovine anaplasmosis is an infectious non-contagious disease transmitted mainly by ticks or fomites contaminated with *Anaplasma marginale*. Once cattle have developed the disease it can be treated with antibiotics or chemotherapy, although with partial success. Still, there is no effective and global prophylactic method available, mainly because of variability and diversity showed by different *A. marginale* strains distributed worldwide. In this regard, several proteins have been proposed as immunogens, MSPs, OMPs, Type IV Secretion System Proteins and some other hypothetical proteins, which have been chosen either by experimental evidence or more recently by genome-based analysis. So far, the results suggest that a single molecule will not be enough to trigger a protective immune response in the host, so it is necessary to identify other proteins or epitopes with adequate immunological properties, a process in which omics tools have potential. In order to develop a vaccine against bovine anaplasmosis, it has been proposed by the use of combinations of molecules, exposure formats and application protocols to provide an effective control of the disease.

Keywords: *Anaplasma marginale*, genomics, vaccinology, bovine anaplasmosis, OMP, MSP

1. Introduction

Tick-borne diseases are considered a major obstacle and the cause of great economic impact for livestock production [1]. Control measures currently available for tick-borne diseases include the use of acaricides for reduction or tick populations, specific chemotherapy, chemoprophylaxis, controlled exposure and vaccination. These measures limit losses caused by ticks and the diseases they transmit [2]. Globally, the most important rickettsial disease in cattle is bovine anaplasmosis caused by *Anaplasma marginale* [3].

Vaccination is the method of choice for preventing infectious diseases. In the case of bovine anaplasmosis, while there are live vaccines, these pose many risks, including: (*i*) spread of other blood-borne pathogens, such as *Babesia* spp. and virus-like bovine leukemia virus to mention a few [4]; (*ii*) standardization of vaccine dose; (*iii*) maintenance of carrier animals; (*iv*) quality control and production; (*v*) maintenance and transportation of vaccines to the end user, including the need of a cold chain [5, 6].

Inactivated vaccines based on the use of the extracted bacteria while effective, are restricted due to: (*i*) potential contamination with erythrocyte membrane antigens; (*ii*) wide antigenic variation between *Anaplasma* strains [7]; (*iii*) possible short-term immunity; and (iv) amelioration of clinical signs while not preventing infection, so the animals remain carriers for the rest of their lives [8].

Vaccine design is compounded by the large antigenic and genetic diversity found in strains from a region to another, within the same herd and even within the same animal [9, 10]. Current investigations focus on the search for new alternatives for designing vaccines and diagnostic assays [11–13]. In this review, besides discussing some fundamental aspects of anaplasmosis, we focus on the molecular characteristics that make *A. marginale* capable to persist in nature including: (*i*) the mechanisms of evasion of the host's immune response; (*ii*) diversity; (*iii*) hypervariability of some of its components; or (*iv*) replication.

2. The causal agent

Anaplasma marginale is a tick-borne pathogen and the causative agent of bovine anaplasmosis [14]. *A. marginale* is classified in the Rickettsial order, reorganized into two families such as Anaplasmataceae and Rickettsiaceae [15]. *Anaplasma* organisms are obligate intracellular Gram-negative rickettsia, found exclusively within vacuoles derived from the erythrocyte membrane, and are membrane-bound within the cytoplasm of the host cell. *A. marginale* persist in nature in mammalian and ticks hosts, which serve as reservoirs of infection [16]. In the bovine, *A. marginale* infect erythrocytes and endothelial cells [17]. The infection process in endothelial cell has not been described and it is considered as of no relevance within the persistence mechanisms for the rickettsia [18]. Ticks transmit rickettsia from the salivary glands during feeding (**Figure 1**), and within the erythrocyte, the rickettsia replicates by binary fission to form 8–12 initial bodies and exit from the erythrocyte does not involve destruction of the host's cell [19]. Once out of the host cell, the initial bodies invade new erythrocytes in endless cycles. Ticks acquires the rickettsia while feeding on carrier hosts. In the tick, the rickettsia infects midgut cells, where there is a first cycle of replication and from here dense forms move to other tissues. After several rounds of replication, dense forms travel to the salivary glands where the rickettsia is transmitted to a new mammalian host [16, 20].

http://dx.doi.org/10.5772/intechopen.72637

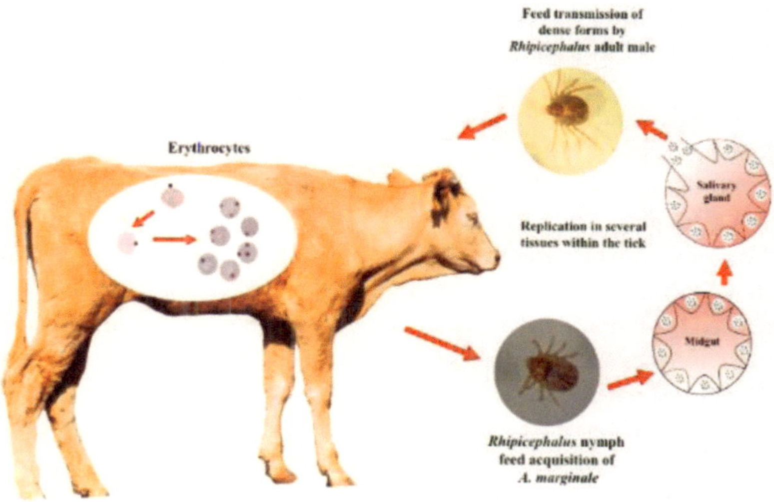

Figure 1. Proposed life cycle of *A. marginale* in bovine. Modified from [20].

Many species of ticks have been implicated in the transmission of *A. marginale,* although *Dermacentor andersoni* is the most studied of all [16]. Recent studies have focused on the role of ticks *Rhipicephalus* (*Boophilus*) *microplus* as vectors of bovine anaplasmosis, an issue discussed below [21, 22].

The first *A. marginale* sequenced genome published [23] present a very complete description of the known features to that date. Up to now, there are at least 2 full genome sequences published (St. Maries and Florida), other 2 almost complete sequences, and 10 more partially annotated sequences (NCBI/Genome). Comparative studies with the available genome sequences have been carried out with very interesting results as far as the study of hypervariable genes/antigens [24], while other genome/transcriptome analysis have focused on the transmission phenotype genes involved [25].

In this chapter, we will review the information available, since the publication of the St. Maries genome to the specific genes that have been studied as vaccine candidates. Vaccination against bovine Anaplasmosis traditionally relied on attenuated [5, 26] and inactivated organisms [6, 27]. Both of these types of vaccines will, in most cases, induce a degree of immunity, which do not prevent infection. There are a number of examples of experimental vaccines, but in this review only those cases where there has been modification of the organism or recombinant antigens are included as vaccine candidates will be discussed.

2.1. Major surface proteins as vaccine candidates

Over the last 30 years, six neutralization-sensitive membrane-exposed proteins were originally reported in 1984 [28, 29] and later named **M**ajor **S**urface **P**roteins [30]. This group of proteins has been the subject of a great number of studies aimed at developing a vaccine.

Msp1 is a heterodimer composed by Msp1a (100 kDa) and Msp1b (105 kDa) joined in a non-covalent manner and are exposed on the surface of *A. marginale* [31]. Details of the genetics, structure, and composition of these two peptides have been described elsewhere [24]. Msp1a is coded by a single gene and its product is composed of a variable number of tandem-repeat units of 28–32 aa in length at the amino terminus. The carboxyl end is conserved and extends mostly as an intracellular domain [32]. Msp1b is coded by a multigene family that expresses several variants during the acute and chronic phases of the infection [33]. Msp1 is an adhesin toward erythrocytes and tick-gut cells whereas Msp1b only toward bovine erythrocytes [34, 35]. It is now known that the adhesion function in Msp1a is located in the variable region which is composed of several short amino acid sequences (repeats). Analysis of Msp1a repeats from different isolates has shown no association between tick-transmission capabilities and the type or number of repeats present within this variable region [36]. Repeat sequences though have been used for defining genotypes associated to other markers such as the pseudogenes present in Msp2 [37] or distinguishing genotypes in cattle superinfected with two or more different *Anaplasma* strains [10, 38, 39].

Bioinformatic analysis carried out with Msp1a amino acid sequence have shown that Msp1a variable region is rich in highly immunogenic B cell epitopes, yet these sequences are considered distracters to the immune system of the host, despite the fact specific monoclonal antibodies neutralize infection to both the erythrocytes and tick cells [40]. Msp1a also contains Th1 cell epitopes in the carboxyl conserved region, which may be involved in immunoprotection [41]. Initial immunization experiments with recombinant Msp1a showed that autologous immunity was afforded; yet heterologous immunity was poor [42]. In a semi-controlled experiment where Msp1a was used as marker for matching the vaccine strain and the local strain in an inactivated vaccine trial in the field, which resulted in partial immunity except when the challenge was carried with the autologous strain but not when challenge was carried with heterologous Msp1a-matched strains [7].

More recently, two epitopes, STSSQL (Am1), located within the consensus sequence of the repeat and SEASTSSQLGA (Am2), which is located in C-terminal end of the 28-aa repetitive motif of the MSP1a protein, were identified using phage display technology for identification of immunodominant epitopes recognized by a neutralizing monoclonal antibody against MSP1a; these peptides were recognized by many but not all healthy infected animals tested by ELISA assay [43]. These synthetic peptides were conjugated to bovine serum albumin and used for immunization of mice, which the authors claim were infected with *A. marginale* was achieved. Details of the challenge strain used in this experiment are absent [44] and there have been no follow-up articles using the same peptides in cattle.

The inclusion of Msp1a or its "conserved epitopes" should be carried with caution as the diversity of this marker is wider in regions where the tick vector is *R. microplus* than in its absence [10, 45]. Vaccination based on Msp1a epitopes is further confounded by the fact that the Msp1a variable region may contain one or several repeats which may include the same or different repeats and that there are more than 300 repeats reported [45, 46] and this number is bound to increase as the number of epidemiology studies is published. Furthermore, the number of Msp1a-distinct strains (up to nine) within the same herd or even within the same animal [10, 47, 48] complicates even more the design of an effective vaccine.

While the adhesion function of Msp1a protein is located on the variable region, number or type of different Msp1a repeat sequences has not been associated with tick-transmission phenotype [49, 50]. Repeat sequences though have been used for defining genotypes associated to other markers such as the pseudogenes present in Msp2 [37] or distinguishing genotypes in cattle superinfected with two or more different *Anaplasma* strains [10, 38, 39].

As for Msp1b, initial experiments indicated that it was a poor immunogen [51, 52]. Further evidence indicates that immunization of naive calves with a recombinant fraction containing the Msp1a-T cell epitopes linked to recombinant Msp1b1, induced a much greater antibody titer to Msp1b than what was previously observed [52, 53].

DNA vaccines based on either one of Msp1a or Msp1b have given disappointing results. In an early effort using a construction pVCL/MSP1a for the immunization of mice and cattle [54], a predominant IgG1 antibody pattern was observed in the two immunized calves. No challenge was performed, however, as it has been proven, an IgG2 response is necessary in order to achieve protection [11, 55]. In a similar study with an Msp1b DNA construct, immunization not only did not induce immunity but immunized animals developed more severe clinical disease than controls [56]. These latter authors did not test for the type of immunoglobulin induced by vaccination.

Further studies with DNA vaccines constructs which included bovine herpes virus 1 tegument protein, BVP22 domain and an invariant-chain major histocompatibility complex class II-targeting motif capable of enhancing dendritic cell antigen uptake and presentation were fused to a sequence encoding a B and T cell antigen from the *A. marginale* Msp1a [57, 58]. This approach included the intradermal inoculation with a mixture of 2 mg of DNA encoding the molecular adjuvants bovine FLT3L and GM-CSF to recruit DCs to the intradermal immunization site, the results of this experiment were very encouraging as they stimulated the desired type of immune response with rapid recall of antibody production over a reasonable period after a single immunization. This study, however, suffers of several flaws (i) the inoculation in different points of the dendritic cells stimulant and the vaccine itself, (ii) while the responses as measured, were in all senses the appropriate ones for resistance, there was no challenge of vaccinated animals and second, the age of the vaccines would not allow for distinction between a solid immune response induced by vaccination or natural resistance commonly observed in animals under 1 year of age [3].

Msp2 is a highly immunodominant 36 kDa protein coded by a multigene family consisting of a functional gene that codes for the amino and carboxyl ends and a variable number of pseudogenes (5 in the St. Maries strain) [59] which recombine with the main gene, through gene conversion, in a single expression site such that the protein is expressed as a new variant in each cycle of rickettsemia, every 6–8 weeks [60]. *msp2* pseudogenes code for hypervariable, hydrophilic sequences containing highly immunogenic B cell epitopes which induce a new immune response consequent to a new Msp2 variant [61]. The amino and carboxyl ends of the protein are hydrophobic conserved segments inserted into the membrane of the rickettsia [62] (and contain Th1 cell type epitopes that are preserved along different geographic strains) [29, 55].

Just like Msp1 and Msp1b, Msp2 was discovered through the neutralization of infection by specific monoclonal antibodies and it was considered a vaccine candidate [28], this has not been the case. While the hypervariable region of the protein contains a number of highly immunogenic type B cell epitopes, it has been recognized that antibody directed to these epitopes are distractors of the immune response during the periodical appearance of Msp2 variants [60, 63].

Msp3 is a very immunogenic 86 k Da protein located on the surface of the rickettsia [28]. *msp3* is also composed by a central hypervariable region coded by several pseudogenes which recombine with the conserved amino and carboxyl ends [64, 65]. Based on previous studies [64] and analysis of the published genome sequence, it is speculated that MSP2 and MSP3 originated from a common ancestor [66], and have diverged since that event. Sequence identity between *msp3* and *msp2* pseudogenes is reduced, an average of 38%, identity within *msp3* pseudogenes 68% and, within *msp2* pseudogenes 78% [66, 67]. Immunologically, Msp2 and Msp3 share epitopes recognized in vitro by $CD4^+$ cells clones from vaccinated cattle [55]. Recombination of pseudogenes in a mosaic pattern also adds to the presentation of polymorphic antigens that, when resolved through 2D electrophoresis, are observed as a series of antigens with the same molecular weight and different but very close isoelectric points [68]. Appearance of Msp2 and Msp3 variants in the persistently infected bovine gives rise to a more complex situation with negative implications for immune protection. Though Msp3 induces production of large amounts of antibodies [69], protection afforded is very limited [70]. Msp3 is known to cross-react with other rickettsiae such as *A. ovis, Ehrlichia risticii, E. wengii, E. equi* and *E. ruminantium*, which make it unsuitable for specific *A. marginale* sero-diagnosis [71].

Msp4 is a 31 kDa protein, encoded by single highly conserved gene, *msp4* [72]. Msp4 is also present in *A. marginale* subsp. *centrale* with 83% identity in the nucleotide sequences and 91.7% in the amino acid level [73]. To date, there is no solid evidence that Msp4 may be involved in protection as, initial studies showed lack of recognition by sera of animals immunized with an initial body membrane fraction [42], however when animals are immunized with a recombinant Msp4 adjuvated with Iscometrix as adjuvant, there seems to induce an antibody response. *msp4* has been used as a base for phylogenetic studies which have shown that there are variations in 168 bp and, of these, 39 bp show utility in parsimony analysis such that isolates from several countries in the Americas can be grouped according to their geographic location [50]. Msp4 is highly conserved over several Mexican isolates [9].

Msp5 is a highly conserved 19 kDa MW protein in *A. marginale, A. marginale* subsp. *centrale* and *A. phagocytophilum* [23, 73–75]. Immunization with Msp5 induces the production of large quantities of non-protective antibodies [69] so it is no suitable for vaccination. Animals naturally infected with the rickettsia produce specific antibodies that can be found in recent and old infections so the protein has been used successfully in a diagnostic competitive-ELISA test [76]. Despite the cross-reaction of antibody between *A. marginale* and *A. marginale* subsp. *centrale* at the competitive-ELISA [74, 77], the test has been adopted as the standard for serologic diagnostic of bovine anaplasmosis.

2.2. Type IV secretion system proteins

Secretion systems in bacteria are complex structures by which they communicate with its environment. There are several secretion systems some which span both the inner membrane (IM) and the outer membrane (OM), and those that span the OM [78]. Among several secretion systems described in nature, type 4 secretion systems (T4SSs) have the unique ability to mediate translocation of DNA (in addition to proteins) into bacterial or eukaryotic target cells. T4SSs are found in both Gram-negative and Gram-positive bacteria and also in some archaea [79]. Their most common role is to mediate the conjugation of plasmid DNA; thus, these systems contribute to the spread of plasmid-borne antibiotic resistance genes. As the ability to conjugate is a common bacterial trait, T4SSs are the most ubiquitous secretion systems in nature. In addition, T4SSs are involved in bacterial pathogenesis in a few organisms, and they mediate the secretion of transforming proteins in *Helicobacter pylori*, toxins in *Bordetella pertussis* and other effector proteins required to support an intracellular lifestyle in bacteria such as *Legionella pneumophila* [79].

Along with the publication of the first complete genome of *A. marginale*, and its annotation, some real or putative homologous genes of T4SS were described in St. Maries genome [23]. Although many studies have been done about MSPs, so far, we still require other approaches to find better vaccine candidates. An approach was shotgun sequencing of the proteins of a membrane-enriched fraction of *A. marginale*, which induced an antibody response in naive calves [80]. In this study, 25 immunoblot positive spots were sequenced and identified through their annotation in the genome. Among the proteins identified VirB9, VirB10 and conjugal transfer protein (CTP), were shown to stimulate an antibody response. Further studies using the same membrane-enriched fractions for the immunization of young cattle showed that their antibodies (IgG2) and Th cells reacted with the recombinant versions of CTP, VirB9 and VirB10 proteins [12]. In a more sophisticated study using far-Western blotting to identify protein linkage between possible antigenic proteins, it was shown that VirB proteins, VirB9-1, VirB9-2 and Virb10 when physically linked, could stimulate a more specific and stronger immune response than when used individually [81]. While presence of B cell epitopes is important in any protein to be used as vaccine candidate, Th cell epitopes are also important as their presence might determine the actual potential use of any antigen in a vaccine. An interesting study, takes synthetic overlapping peptides from VirB9-1, VirB9-2 and VirB10 to test for the presence of such epitopes [82]. T cells from six different MHC Class-II phenotypes outer membrane fraction immunized animals were tested and as expected, it was observed that not all animals reacted with peptides from all three TFSS proteins. While all six animals reacted to the membrane fraction which contained all three VirB9-1, VirB9-2 and VirB10, some animals did not react against rVirB9–1, others reacted poorly against rVirB9-2 or rVirB10 or against only one or two of the overlapping synthetic peptides [82]. The differences in response of T cells from these animals are explained in the context of the Class-II MHC molecules involved in presentation of the epitopes. Interestingly, these authors restricted themselves to Holstein cattle as the subjects to their studies yet, at least in Mexico and other Latin American countries, Holstein cattle are used for milk production and most of them are reared under conditions which preclude the contact with ticks.

These studies clearly show that an immune response that fills the criteria for protection as described is induced [11, 55], these authors though, fall short of proving that the induced immunity is protective as there was no actual confrontation with the virulent live agent. In a different study recombinant VirB9, Virb10 and Elongation Factor Tu (EF-Tu) were tested against the sera of immunoprotected animals naturally infected with two *A. marginale* isolates [83]. These works showed that while all experimentally infected cattle with the autologous isolate had relevant antibodies (IgG2) against VirB9, VirB10 and EF-Tu, only 87% of the animals naturally infected with a heterologous isolate reacted with the recombinant protein by ELISA.

2.3. Outer membrane proteins

The outer membrane of bacteria delimits its structure and is the interface with the host cell. Outer membrane proteins (OMPs) are key components of Gram-negative bacteria and because are involved in adhesion and infection processes they are targeted on vaccine development.

Some effective attempts have been achieved using whole membrane fractions as immunogens against bacterial diseases and due to their relevance OMPs from several pathogens have been extensively studied and proposed as vaccine component. It is known that in addition to composition, OMPs show diversity in function too, but they share structural patterns. Usually, regions with antigenic properties are located on the extracellular loops and show variable composition, meanwhile residues in the transmembrane β-barrel show the highest conservation [61, 84–86]. However, the use of individual components has only been partially successful [86–92], although, it appears that the most relevant OMP antigens have not yet been identified.

High-throughput sequencing technologies are currently available and allow the identification of several genes with potential important functions in the metabolism of the pathogen or in the interaction with its surroundings. For example, from the complete genome of *Anaplasma marginale* [23], the existence of additional outer membrane protein has been elucidated. Additionally, to Msp2 and Msp3, new members of pfam01617 family have been identified, and designated as Omp 1-14. *omp2, omp3* and *omp6* genes are not transcribed in *A. marginale*-infected erythrocytes, tick midgut and salivary glands, and the IDE8 tick cell line, while OMPs 1, 4, 7, 8, 9 and 11 were confirmed to be differentially expressed as proteins in those cell types [93]. Unlike Msp2 and Msp3, these OMPs exhibit high conservation at sequence level as seen in the follow-up of the infection and in comparative analyses with the St. Maries and Florida strain genomes, which increases the possibility of choosing molecules capable of inducing a protective immune response against bovine Anaplasmosis. Omp7 to Omp9 appear as tandem repeats with almost 75% amino acid identity, Omp10 is related to Omp7 to Omp9 with ~ 30% residues identity and Omp6 is a truncated and it is not expressed version of Omp10. Omp7 to Omp9 are part of protective outer membrane fraction and are highly expressed than Omp10 [23, 25, 93, 94].

In spite of the fact that none of these molecules has induced protection when is applied as an individual protein, the importance of OMPs in protective immune response induction has been revealed above all as complexes or associated with a membrane environment.

For example, protection against *Leptospira* was reached using OmpL1 and LipL41 expressed simultaneously in the context of the *E. coli* membrane but, immunization with either membrane-associated protein or as part of a mixture of non-membrane-associated proteins was not protective [53, 95].

These results confirm the importance of OMPs in the infection process and the generation of a protective immune response against pathogens and also reveal the interactions between OMPs and other proteins as well as with their environment. However, production, solubilization and purification of membrane-associated recombinant proteins is not easily achieved [96].

2.4. Hypothetical proteins

Genomic analyses of *A. marginale* have allowed identification of novel annotated proteins whose function has not yet been determined, however, *in silico* analysis and predictions may provide unrevealed information about immunogenic potential.

Some hypothetical proteins have been identified by structure prediction of β-barrel outer membrane and orthology and bioinformatic analysis, such as Am1108, Am127, Am216, Am202, Am936, Am854, Am368, Am854, Am1041, Am109 and Am1096. Some of these proteins have been evaluated as recombinant molecules and recognized by IgG from immunized animals with outer membranes protein, in this case, Am1108 and Am216 elicited specific T cell response proliferation [13, 97]. On the other hand, cattle immunized with recombinant Am854 or Am936 developed higher bacteremia as compared to adjuvant-only controls and outer membrane vaccinates after challenge [13].

The absence of a protective immune response after application of recombinant proteins presumably exposed to *A. marginale,* and therefore, with antigenic characteristics still seems to be insufficient to develop prophylactic methods against bovine anaplasmosis.

Although genomic analyses have revealed valuable information about the composition of *A. marginale*, it will be necessary to complement this knowledge with experimental evidence based in other methods, such as proteomic and transcriptomic tools.

Acknowledgements

Authors thank financial support to projects SEP-CONACYT 161618 granted to SDR and INIFAP SIGI 11343533011 granted to IAE.

Author details

Itzel Amaro-Estrada and Sergio D. Rodríguez-Camarillo*

*Address all correspondence to: rodriguez.sergio@inifap.gob.mx

Anaplasmosis Unit, National Center for Disciplinary Research in Veterinary Parasitology, CENID-PAVET, INIFAP, Jiutepec, Morelos, México

References

[1] Jonsson NN, Bock RE, Jorgensen WK. Productivity and health effects of anaplasmosis and babesiosis on Bos Indicus cattle and their crosses, and the effects of differing intensity of tick control in Australia. Veterinary Parasitology. 2008;**155**(1–2):1-9

[2] Kocan KM, de la Fuente J, Blouin EF. Advances toward understanding the molecular biology of the Anaplasma-tick interface. Frontiers in Bioscience. 2008;**13**:7032-7045

[3] Aubry P, Geale DW. A review of bovine anaplasmosis. Transboundary and Emerging Diseases. 2011;**58**(1):1-30

[4] Rogers R, Dimmock CK, de Vos AJ, Rodwell BJ. Bovine leucosis virus contamination of a vaccine produced in vivo against bovine babesiosis and anaplasmosis. Australian Veterinary Journal. 1988;**65**(9):285-287. Available from: http://dx.doi.org/10.1111/j.1751-0813.1988.tb16144.x

[5] Abdala AA, Pipano E, Aguirre DH, Gaido AB, Zurbriggen MA, Mangold AJ, et al. Frozen and fresh Anaplasma centrale vaccines in the protection of cattle against *Anaplasma marginale* infection. Revue d'Élevage et de Médecine Vétérinaire des Pays Tropicaux. 1990;**43**(2):155-158

[6] Rodríguez SD, Garcîa Ortiz MA, Hernández Salgado G, Santos Cerda NA, Aboytes Torre R, Cantó Alarcón GJ. *Anaplasma marginale* inactivated vaccine: Dose titration against a homologous challenge. Comparative Immunology, Microbiology and Infectious Diseases. 2000;**23**(4):239-252

[7] Ocampo Espinoza V, Vázquez JES, Aguilar MD, Ortiz MÁG, Alarcón GJC, Rodríguez SD. *Anaplasma marginale*: Lack of cross-protection between strains that share MSP1a variable region and MSP4. Veterinary Microbiology. 2006;**114**(1–2):34-40. Available from: http://www.sciencedirect.com/science/article/pii/S037811350500444X

[8] Reinbold JB, Coetzee JF, Hollis LC, Nickell JS, Riegel CM, Christopher JA, et al. Comparison of iatrogenic transmission of *Anaplasma marginale* in Holstein steers via needle and needle-free injection techniques. American Journal of Veterinary Research. 2010;**71**(10):1178-1188

[9] Jiménez-Ocampo R, Vega y Murguía CA, Oviedo N, Rojas Ramírez EE, García-Ortiz MA, Preciado de la Torre JF, et al. Diversidad genética de la región variable de los genes msp1a y msp4 en cepas de *Anaplasma marginale* de México genetic diversity of the msp1a gene variable region and msp4 gene of *Anaplasma marginale* strains from Mexico. Revista Mexicana de Ciencias Pecuarias. 2012;**3**(3):373-387

[10] Castañeda-Ortiz EJ, Ueti MW, Camacho-Nuez M, Mosqueda JJ, Mousel MR, Johnson WC, et al. Association of *Anaplasma marginale* strain superinfection with infection prevalence within tropical regions. PLoS One. 2015;**10**(3):e0120748. Available from: http://dx.plos.org/10.1371/journal.pone.0120748

[11] Barigye R, García-Ortiz MA, Rojas Ramírez EE, Rodríguez SD. Identification of IgG2-specific antigens in Mexican *Anaplasma marginale* strains. Annals of the New York Academy of Sciences. 2004;**1026**:84-94

[12] Lopez JE, Palmer GH, Brayton KA, Dark MJ, Leach SE, Brown WC. Immunogenicity of *Anaplasma marginale* type IV secretion system proteins in a protective outer membrane vaccine. Infection and Immunity. 2007;**75**(5):2333-2342. Available from: http://www.ncbi.nlm.nih.gov/pmc/articles/PMC1865776/

[13] Ducken DR, Brown WC, Alperin DC, Brayton KA, Reif KE, Turse JE, et al. Subdominant outer membrane antigens in *Anaplasma marginale*: Conservation, antigenicity, and protective capacity using recombinant protein. PLoS One. 2015;**10**(6):e0129309. Available from: http://dx.plos.org/10.1371/journal.pone.0129309

[14] Ristic M. Anaplasmosis. In: Diseases of Cattle in the Tropics. Dordrecht: Springer Netherlands; 1981. pp. 327-344

[15] Dumler JS, Barbet AF, Bekker CP, Dasch GA, Palmer GH, Ray SC, et al. Reorganization of genera in the families Rickettsiaceae and Anaplasmataceae in the order Rickettsiales: Unification of some species of Ehrlichia with Anaplasma, Cowdria with Ehrlichia and Ehrlichia with Neorickettsia, descriptions of six new species combinations and designation of Ehrlichia equi and "HGE agent" as subjective synonyms of Ehrlichia phagocytophila. International Journal of Systematic and Evolutionary Microbiology. 2001;**51**(Pt 6):2145-2165

[16] Kocan KM, de la Fuente J, Blouin EF, Coetzee JF, S a E. The natural history of *Anaplasma marginale*. Veterinary Parasitology. 2010;**167**(2–4):95-107

[17] Carreño AD, Alleman AR, Barbet AF, Palmer GH, Noh SM, Johnson CM. *In vivo* endothelial cell infection by *Anaplasma marginale*. Veterinary Pathology. 2007;**44**(1):116-118

[18] Wamsley HL, Alleman AR, Johnson CM, Barbet AF, Abbott JR. Investigation of endothelial cells as an in vivo nidus of *Anaplasma marginale* infection in cattle. Veterinary Microbiology. 2011;**153**(3–4):264-273

[19] Kessler RH, Ristic M. In vitro cultivation of *Anaplasma marginale*: Invasion of and development in noninfected erythrocytes. American Journal of Veterinary Research. 1979;**40**(12):1774-1776

[20] Rodríguez SD, García Ortiz MÁ, Jiménez Ocampo R, Vega y Murguía CA. Molecular epidemiology of bovine anaplasmosis with a particular focus in Mexico. Infection, Genetics and Evolution. 2009;**9**(6):1092-1101

[21] Futse JE, Ueti MW, Knowles DP, Palmer GH. Transmission of *Anaplasma marginale* by Boophilus Microplus: Retention of vector competence in the absence of vector-pathogen interaction. Journal of Clinical Microbiology. 2003;**41**(8):3829-3834

[22] Ruiz PMG, Passos LMF, Ribeiro MFB. Lack of infectivity of a Brazilian *Anaplasma marginale* isolate for *Boophilus microplus* ticks. Veterinary Parasitology. 2005;**128**(3–4):325-331

[23] Brayton KA, Kappmeyer LS, Herndon DR, Dark MJ, Tibbals DL, Palmer GH, et al. Complete genome sequencing of *Anaplasma marginale* reveals that the surface is skewed to two superfamilies of outer membrane proteins. Proceedings of the National Academy of Sciences of the United States of America. 2005;**102**(3):844-849

[24] Dark MJ, Al-Khedery B, Barbet AF. Multistrain genome analysis identifies candidate vaccine antigens of *Anaplasma marginale*. Vaccine. 2011;**29**(31):4923-4932

[25] Pierlé SA, Dark MJ, Dahmen D, Palmer GH, Brayton KA. Comparative genomics and transcriptomics of trait-gene association. BMC Genomics. 2012;**13**:669. Available from: http://www.pubmedcentral.nih.gov/articlerender.fcgi?artid=3542260&tool=pmcentrez&rendertype=abstract

[26] Ristic M, Carson CA. Methods of immunoprophylaxis against bovine anaplasmosis with emphasis on use of the attenuated *Anaplasma marginale* vaccine. Advances in Experimental Medicine and Biology. 1977;**93**:151-188

[27] Wilson JS, Trace JC. A new inactivated vaccine for bovine anaplasmosis. Bulletin - Office International Des Epizooties. 1966;**66**(1):897-902

[28] Palmer GH, McGuire TC. Immune serum against *Anaplasma marginale* initial bodies neutralizes infectivity for cattle. Journal of Immunology. 1984;**133**(2):1010-1015

[29] McGuire TC, Palmer GH, Goff WL, Johnson MI, Davis WC. Common and isolate-restricted antigens of *Anaplasma marginale* detected with monoclonal antibodies. Infection and Immunity. 1984;**45**(3):697-700

[30] Palmer GH, Kocan KM, Barron SJ, Hair JA, Barbet AF, Davis WC, et al. Presence of common antigens, including major surface protein epitopes, between the cattle (intraerythrocytic) and tick stages of *Anaplasma marginale*. Infection and Immunity. 1985;**50**(3):881-886

[31] Barbet AF, Palmer GH, Myler PJ, McGuire TC. Characterization of an immunoprotective protein complex of *Anaplasma marginale* by cloning and expression of the gene coding for polypeptide Am105L. Infection and Immunity. 1987;**55**(10):2428-2435

[32] Allred DR, McGuire TC, Palmer GH, Leib SR, Harkins TM, McElwain TF, et al. Molecular basis for surface antigen size polymorphisms and conservation of a neutralization-sensitive epitope in *Anaplasma marginale*. Proceedings of the National Academy of Sciences of the United States of America. 1990;**87**(8):3220-3224. Available from: http://www.ncbi.nlm.nih.gov/pmc/articles/PMC53867/

[33] Viseshakul N, Kamper S, Bowie MV, Barbet AF. Sequence and expression analysis of a surface antigen gene family of the rickettsia *Anaplasma marginale*. Gene. 2000;**253**(1):45-53

[34] McGarey DJ, Allred DR. Characterization of hemagglutinating components on the *Anaplasma marginale* initial body surface and identification of possible adhesins. Infection and Immunity. 1994;**62**(10):4587-4593

[35] McGarey DJ, Barbet AF, Palmer GH, McGuire TC, Allred DR. Putative adhesins of *Anaplasma marginale*: Major surface polypeptides 1a and 1b. Infection and Immunity. 1994;**62**(10):4594-4601

[36] Cabezas-Cruz A, Passos LMF, Lis K, Kenneil R, Valdes JJ, Ferrolho J, et al. Functional and immunological relevance of *Anaplasma marginale* major surface protein 1a sequence and structural analysis. PLoS One. 2013;**8**(6)

[37] Palmer GH, Futse JE, Leverich CK, Knowles DP, Rurangirwa FR, Brayton KA. Selection for simple major surface protein 2 variants during *Anaplasma marginale* transmission to immunologically naïve animals. Infection and Immunity. 2007;**75**(3):1502-1506

[38] Futse JE, Brayton KA, Dark MJ, Knowles DP, Palmer GH. Superinfection as a driver of genomic diversification in antigenically variant pathogens. Proceedings of the National Academy of Sciences of the United States of America. 2008;**105**(6):2123-2127

[39] Leverich CK, Palmer GH, Knowles DP, Brayton KA. Tick-borne transmission of two genetically distinct *Anaplasma marginale* strains following superinfection of the mammalian reservoir host. Infection and Immunity. 2008;**76**(9):4066-4070

[40] Palmer GH, Waghela SD, Barbet AF, Davis WC, McGuire TC. Characterization of a neutralization-sensitive epitope on the am 105 surface protein of *Anaplasma marginale*. International Journal for Parasitology. 1987;**17**(7):1279-1285

[41] Brown WC, McGuire TC, Mwangi W, Kegerreis KA, Macmillan H, Lewin HA, et al. Major histocompatibility complex class II DR-restricted memory CD4(+) T lymphocytes recognize conserved immunodominant epitopes of *Anaplasma marginale* major surface protein 1a. Infection and Immunity. 2002;**70**(10):5521-5532

[42] Tebele N, Palmer GH. Crossprotective immunity between the Florida and a Zimbabwe stock of *Anaplasma marginale*. Tropical Animal Health and Production. 1991;**23**(4):197-202

[43] Santos PS, Nascimento R, Rodrigues LP, Santos FAA, Faria PCB, Martins JRS, et al. Functional epitope core motif of the *Anaplasma marginale* major surface protein 1a and its incorporation onto bioelectrodes for antibody detection. PLoS One. 2012;**7**(3):e33045

[44] Santos PS, Sena AAS, Nascimento R, Araújo TG, Mendes MM, Martins JRS, et al. Epitope-based vaccines with the *Anaplasma marginale* MSP1a functional motif induce a balanced humoral and cellular immune response in mice. PLoS One. 2013;**8**(4):1-9

[45] Quiroz-Castañeda RE, Amaro-Estrada I, Rodríguez-Camarillo SD. *Anaplasma marginale*: Diversity, virulence, and vaccine landscape through a genomics approach. BioMed Research International. 2016;**2016**:9032085. Available from: http://www.ncbi.nlm.nih.gov/pmc/articles/PMC5005611/

[46] Cabezas-Cruz A, de la Fuente J. *Anaplasma marginale* major surface protein 1a: A marker of strain diversity with implications for control of bovine anaplasmosis. Ticks and Tick-borne Diseases. 2015;**6**(3):205-210

[47] Palmer GH, Knowles DP, Rodriguez J-L, Gnad DP, Hollis LC, Marston T, et al. Stochastic transmission of multiple genotypically distinct *Anaplasma marginale* strains in a herd with high prevalence of anaplasma infection. Journal of Clinical Microbiology. 2004;**42**(11):5381-5384. Available from: http://www.ncbi.nlm.nih.gov/pmc/articles/PMC525272/

[48] Ybañez AP, Ybañez RHD, Claveria FG, Cruz-Flores MJ, Xuenan X, Yokoyama N, et al. High genetic diversity of *Anaplasma marginale* detected from Philippine cattle. The Journal of Veterinary Medical Science. 2014;**76**(7):1009-1014. Available from: http://www.ncbi.nlm.nih.gov/pubmed/24717413

[49] de la Fuente J, Garcia-Garcia JC, Blouin EF, Kocan KM. Characterization of the functional domain of major surface protein 1a involved in adhesion of the rickettsia *Anaplasma marginale* to host cells. Veterinary Microbiology. 2003;**91**(2–3):265-283

[50] de la Fuente J, Ruybal P, Mtshali MS, Naranjo V, Shuqing L, Mangold AJ, et al. Analysis of world strains of *Anaplasma marginale* using major surface protein 1a repeat sequences. Veterinary Microbiology. 2007;**119**(2–4):382-390 [cited 2016 Jan 4]. Available from: http://www.sciencedirect.com/science/article/pii/S0378113506003828

[51] Palmer GH, Barbet AF, Kuttler KL, McGuire TC. Detection of an *Anaplasma marginale* common surface protein present in all stages of infection. Journal of Clinical Microbiology. 1986;**23**(6):1078-1083

[52] Brown WC, Palmer GH, Lewin HA, McGuire TC. CD4(+) T lymphocytes from calves immunized with *Anaplasma marginale* major surface protein 1 (MSP1), a heteromeric complex of MSP1a and MSP1b, preferentially recognize the MSP1a carboxyl terminus that is conserved among strains. Infection and Immunity. 2001;**69**(11):6853-6862

[53] Macmillan H, Norimine J, Brayton KA, Palmer GH, Brown WC. Physical linkage of naturally complexed bacterial outer membrane proteins enhances immunogenicity. Infection and Immunity. 2008;**76**(3):1223-1229

[54] Arulkanthan A, Brown WC, McGuire TC, Knowles DP. Biased immunoglobulin G1 isotype responses induced in cattle with DNA expressing msp1a of *Anaplasma marginale*. Infection and Immunity. 1999;**67**(7):3481-3487

[55] Brown WC, Shkap V, Zhu D, McGuire TC, Tuo W, McElwain TF, et al. CD4(+) T-lymphocyte and immunoglobulin G2 responses in calves immunized with *Anaplasma marginale* outer membranes and protected against homologous challenge. Infection and Immunity. 1998;**66**(11):5406-5413

[56] de Andrade GM, Machado RZ, Vidotto MC, Vidotto O. Immunization of bovines using a DNA vaccine (pcDNA3.1/MSP1b) prepared from the Jaboticabal strain of *Anaplasma marginale*. Annals of the New York Academy of Sciences 2004;**1026**:257–266

[57] Mwangi W, Brown WC, Splitter GA, Zhuang Y, Kegerreis K, Palmer GH. Enhancement of antigen acquisition by dendritic cells and MHC class II-restricted epitope presentation to CD4+ T cells using VP22 DNA vaccine vectors that promote intercellular spreading following initial transfection. Journal of Leukocyte Biology. 2005;**78**(2):401-411

[58] Mwangi W, Brown WC, Splitter GA, Davies CJ, Howard CJ, Hope JC, et al. DNA vaccine construct incorporating intercellular trafficking and intracellular targeting motifs effectively primes and induces memory B- and T-cell responses in outbred animals. Clinical and Vaccine Immunology. 2007;**14**(3):304-311

[59] Palmer GH, Eid G, Barbet AF, McGuire TC, McElwain TF. The immunoprotective *Anaplasma marginale* major surface protein 2 is encoded by a polymorphic multigene family. Infection and Immunity. 1994;**62**(9):3808-3816

[60] French DM, Brown WC, Palmer GH. Emergence of *Anaplasma marginale* antigenic variants during persistent rickettsemia. Infection and Immunity. 1999;**67**(11):5834-5840

[61] Barbet AF, Lundgren A, Yi J, Rurangirwa FR, Palmer GH. Antigenic variation of *Anaplasma marginale* by expression of MSP2 mosaics. Infection and Immunity. 2000;**68**(11):6133-6138

[62] Noh SM, Brayton KA, Knowles DP, Agnes JT, Dark MJ, Brown WC, et al. Differential expression and sequence conservation of the *Anaplasma marginale* msp2 gene superfamily outer membrane proteins. Infection and Immunity. 2006;**74**(6):3471-3479

[63] Abbott JR, Palmer GH, Howard CJ, Hope JC, Brown WC. *Anaplasma marginale* major surface protein 2 CD4+–T-cell epitopes are evenly distributed in conserved and Hypervariable regions (HVR), whereas linear B-cell epitopes are predominantly located in the HVR. Infection and Immunity. 2004;**72**(12):7360-7366

[64] Alleman AR, Palmer GH, McGuire TC, McElwain TF, Perryman LE, Barbet AF. *Anaplasma marginale* major surface protein 3 is encoded by a polymorphic, multigene family. Infection and Immunity. 1997;**65**(1):156-163

[65] Meeus PFM, Brayton KA, Palmer GH, Barbet AF. Conservation of a gene conversion mechanism in two distantly related paralogues of *Anaplasma marginale*. Molecular Microbiology. 2003;**47**(3):633-643 [cited 2016 Feb 3]. Available from: http://doi.wiley.com/10.1046/j.1365-2958.2003.03331.x

[66] Meeus PF, Barbet AF. Ingenious gene generation. Trends in Microbiology. 2001;**9**(8):353-356

[67] Brayton KA, Knowles DP, McGuire TC, Palmer GH. Efficient use of a small genome to generate antigenic diversity in tick-borne ehrlichial pathogens. Proceedings of the National Academy of Sciences. 2001;**98**(7):4130-4135

[68] Barbet AF, Blentlinger R, Yi J, Lundgren AM, Blouin EF, Kocan KM. Comparison of surface proteins of *Anaplasma marginale* grown in tick cell culture, tick salivary glands, and cattle. Infection and Immunity. 1999;**67**(1):102-107

[69] Palmer GH, McElwain TF. Molecular basis for vaccine development against anaplasmosis and babesiosis. Veterinary Parasitology. 1995;**57**(1–3):233-253

[70] McGuire TC, Davis WC, Brassfield AL, McElwain TF, Palmer GH. Identification of *Anaplasma marginale* long-term carrier cattle by detection of serum antibody to isolated MSP-3. Journal of Clinical Microbiology. 1991;**29**(4):788-793

[71] Alleman AR, Barbet AF. Evaluation of *Anaplasma marginale* major surface protein 3 (MSP3) as a diagnostic test antigen. Journal of Clinical Microbiology. 1996;**34**(2):270-276

[72] Oberle SM, Barbet AF. Derivation of the complete msp4 gene sequence of *Anaplasma marginale* without cloning. Gene. 1993;**136**(1–2):291-294

[73] Molad T, Brayton KA, Palmer GH, Michaeli S, Shkap V. Molecular conservation of MSP4 and MSP5 in *Anaplasma marginale* and A. Centrale vaccine strain. Veterinary Microbiology. 2004;**100**(1–2):55-64

[74] Visser ES, TC MG, Palmer GH, Davis WC, Shkap V, Pipano E, et al. The *Anaplasma marginale* msp5 gene encodes a 19-kilodalton protein conserved in all recognized Anaplasma species. Infection and Immunity. 1992;**60**(12):5139-5144

[75] Strik NI, Alleman AR, Barbet AF, Sorenson HL, Wamsley HL, Gaschen FP, et al. Characterization of *Anaplasma phagocytophilum* major surface protein 5 and the extent of its cross-reactivity with *A. marginale*. Clinical and Vaccine Immunology. 2007;**14**(3):262-268

[76] Torioni de Echaide S, Knowles DP, McGuire TC, Palmer GH, Suarez CE, McElwain TF. Detection of cattle naturally infected with *Anaplasma marginale* in a region of endemicity by nested PCR and a competitive enzyme-linked immunosorbent assay using recombinant major surface protein 5. Journal of Clinical Microbiology. 1998;**36**(3):777-782

[77] Knowles D, Torioni de Echaide S, Palmer G, McGuire T, Stiller D, McElwain T. Antibody against an *Anaplasma marginale* MSP5 epitope common to tick and erythrocyte stages identifies persistently infected cattle. Journal of Clinical Microbiology. 1996;**34**(9):2225-2230

[78] Costa TRD, Felisberto-Rodrigues C, Meir A, Prevost MS, Redzej A, Trokter M, et al. Secretion systems in gram-negative bacteria: Structural and mechanistic insights. Nature Reviews. Microbiology. 2015;**13**(6):343-359

[79] Alvarez-Martinez CE, Christie PJ. Biological diversity of prokaryotic type IV secretion systems. Microbiology and Molecular Biology Reviews. 2009;**73**(4):775-808

[80] Lopez JE, Siems WF, Palmer GH, Brayton KA, McGuire TC, Norimine J, et al. Identification of novel antigenic proteins in a complex *Anaplasma marginale* outer membrane immunogen by mass spectrometry and genomic mapping. Infection and Immunity. 2005;**73**(12): 8109-8118

[81] Morse K, Norimine J, Palmer GH, Sutten EL, Baszler TV, Brown WC. Association and evidence for linked recognition of type IV secretion system proteins VirB9-1, VirB9-2, and VirB10 in *Anaplasma marginale*. Infection and Immunity. 2012;**80**(1):215-227

[82] Morse K, Norimine J, Hope JC, Brown WC. Breadth of the CD4+ T cell response to *Anaplasma marginale* VirB9-1, VirB9-2 and VirB10 and MHC class II DR and DQ restriction elements. Immunogenetics. 2012;**64**(7):507-523. Available from: http://dx.doi.org/10.1007/s00251-012-0606-4

[83] Araújo FR, Costa CM, Ramos CAN, Farias TA, De Souza IIF, Melo ESP, et al. IgG and IgG2 antibodies from cattle naturally infected with *Anaplasma marginale* recognize the recombinant vaccine candidate antigens VirB9, VirB10, and elongation factor-Tu. Memórias do Instituto Oswaldo Cruz. 2008;**103**(2):186-190

[84] Zhang JZ, Guo H, Winslow GM, Yu XJ. Expression of members of the 28-Kilodalton major outer membrane protein family of *Ehrlichia chaffeensis* during persistent infection. Infection and Immunity. 2004;**72**(8):4336-4343

[85] Callaghan MJ, Buckee CO, Jolley KA, Kriz P, Maiden MCJ, Gupta S. The effect of immune selection on the structure of the meningococcal Opa protein repertoire. Guttman DS, editor. PLoS Pathogens. 2008;**4**(3):e1000020

[86] Baldo L, Desjardins CA, Russell JA, Stahlhut JK, Werren JH. Accelerated microevolution in an outer membrane protein (OMP) of the intracellular bacteria Wolbachia. BMC Evolutionary Biology. 2010;**10**:48

[87] Lin J, Huang S, Zhang Q. Outer membrane proteins: Key players for bacterial adaptation in host niches. Microbes and Infection. 2002;**4**(3):325-331

[88] Wang Y, Chen Z, Qiao F, Zhong Z, Xu J, Wang Z, et al. and the outer membrane properties of Brucella melitensis. 2010;**303**:92-100

[89] Brattig NW, Bazzocchi C, Kirschning CJ, Reiling N, Büttner DW, Ceciliani F, et al. The major surface protein of Wolbachia endosymbionts in filarial nematodes elicits immune responses through TLR2 and TLR4. Journal of Immunology. 2004;**173**(1):437-445

[90] Oliveira TL, Grassmann AA, Schuch RA, Clair A. Evaluation of the *Leptospira interrogans* outer membrane protein OmpL37 as a vaccine candidate. PLoS ONE. 2015;**10**(11): e0142821. Available from: https://doi.org/10.1371/journal.pone.0142821

[91] Pan J, Li C, Ye Z. Immunoproteomic approach for screening vaccine candidates from bacterial outer membrane proteins. In: Thomas S, editor. Vaccine Design. Methods in Molecular Biology. 2016;**1404**:519-528. Vaccines for Veterinary Diseases, Volume 2. New York, NY: Humana Press; 2016

[92] Singh R, Garg N, Shukla G, Capalash N, Sharma P, Fernandez MM. Immunoprotective eefficacy of *Acinetobacter baumannii* outer membrane protein, FilF, predicted in silico as a potential vaccine candidate. Frontiers in Microbiology. 2016;**7**(February):1-9

[93] Noh SM, Brayton KA, Knowles DP, Agnes JT, Dark MJ, Brown WC, et al. Differential expression and sequence conservation of the *Anaplasma marginale* msp2 gene superfamily outer membrane proteins. Infection and Immunity. 2006;**74**(6):3471-3479

[94] Crosby FL, Wamsley HL, Pate MG, Lundgren AM, Noh SM, Munderloh UG, et al. Knockout of an outer membrane protein operon of *Anaplasma marginale* by transposon mutagenesis. BMC Genomics. 2014;**15**(1):278. Available from: http://www.ncbi.nlm.nih.gov/pubmed/24725301

[95] Haake DA, Mazel MK, McCoy AM, Milward F, Chao G, Matsunaga J, et al. Leptospiral outer membrane proteins OmpL1 and LipL41 exhibit synergistic immunoprotection. Infection and Immunity 1999;**67**(12):6572-6582

[96] Wen Z, Boddicker MA, Kaufhold RM, Khandelwal P, Durr E, Qiu P, et al. Recombinant expression of chlamydia trachomatis major outer membrane protein in *E. coli* outer membrane as a substrate for vaccine research. BMC Microbiology. 2016:1-13

[97] Nuñez PA, Moretta R, Ruybal P, Wilkowsky S, Farber MD. Immunogenicity of hypothetical highly conserved proteins as novel antigens in *Anaplasma marginale*. Current Microbiology. 2013;**68**(3):269-277. Available from: http://dx.doi.org/10.1007/s00284-013-0475-6

Chapter 4

Genome-Based Vaccinology Applied to Bovine Babesiosis

Juan Mosqueda,
Diego Josimar Hernández-Silva and
Mario Hidalgo-Ruiz

Additional information is available at the end of the chapter

http://dx.doi.org/10.5772/intechopen.72636

Abstract

Genomics approaches in veterinary research have been a very useful tool to identify candidates with potential to be used in prevention of animal diseases. In *Babesia*, genome information analysis has elucidated a wide variety of protein families and some members are described in this chapter. Here, we present some of the most recent studies about *B. bovis* and *B. bigemina* genomes where some proteins have been identified with potential to prevent infections by these parasites.

Keywords: bovine babesiosis, bioinformatics, vaccines, genomics

1. Introduction

Bovine babesiosis is a tick-transmitted disease caused by apicomplexan parasites of the genus *Babesia*. This disease is caused by *Babesia bovis* and *B. bigemina* in the Americas including Mexico, where it is distributed in tropical and subtropical regions, occupying 51.5% of the national territory [1, 2]. This disease was reported for the first time by Viktor Babes in Rumania in 1888. However, it was until 1893 when Smith and Kilborne demonstrated that the disease is transmitted to cattle by infected ticks [3, 4]. In Mexico, the first report of bovine babesiosis occurred in 1905; however, it is believed that it was first introduced to the American continent by the Spaniards during the conquest. To date, measures used to control bovine babesiosis include vector control, an early diagnosis, treatment of sick animals and vaccination. The negative, severe impact that cattle fever tick and babesiosis have in the cattle industry in Mexico and the world has not diminished due mainly to a lack of commercially available, safe and effective vaccines. Vaccines based on approaches using genomics and bioinformatics are a promissory solution to this problem [5]. It has been shown that experimental vaccines based on recombinant antigens have been developed successfully in apicomplexan parasites like *Plasmodium, Toxoplasma* and *Theileria* [6–8]. With the completion of the *B. bovis* genome [9] and the partial sequencing of the *Babesia bigemina* genome (http://www.sanger.ac.uk/), it is now possible to study these pathogens to the genomic level, taking advantage of the bioinformatics tools developed for this purpose. This approach is now generating valuable information on the essential characteristics of the genome structure and allows comparative analyses with genomes of other apicomplexan pathogens of importance in human and animal health, as well as the identification of genes with a potential use in diagnostics, vaccines or therapeutics. More specific analyses are also possible with the generation of expressed sequence tags (EST) obtained for *B. bovis*, which allow the analysis of those genes specifically expressed in the different stages of the parasite's life cycle [10] and, finally, implementation of methods for genome-wide analysis like microarrays which will be in short available for their use [11]. Additionally, research on this important disease is complemented with all the information generated so far about those genes codifying antigens with a potential as candidates in vaccines, diagnostics or therapeutics, which have been discovered in the last 30 years. Equally important is the knowledge about the life cycle of the parasite, the interaction with the vector tick and the genes involved in this interaction, which are poorly studied so far. In the following sections, we describe the most relevant aspects of the *B. bovis* and *B. bigemina* genomes and genes characterized to date.

2. Babesiosis

2.1. *Babesia bovis* genome

Although *Babesia bovis, B. bigemina* and *B. divergens* are causative agents of bovine babesiosis, *B. bovis* is regarded as the most important and has a bigger impact in the livestock industry due to its virulence and high mortality rate. For this reason, the *B. bovis* genome was the first to be sequenced. This was done by Washigton State University in collaboration with the Agricultural Research Service and The Institute for Genomic Research (TIGR) in the USA. The genome sequence was obtained from the T2Bo strain, a virulent strain isolated from a clinical case in Texas, USA.

The genome of *Babesia bovis* has a length of 8.2 Mbp, contains 3671 genes and consists of four chromosomes, three of them are acrocentric: chromosome 1, has a length of 1.25 Mpb, is the smallest and contains a gap, which is estimated to be 150 Kpb long. Chromosome 2 is fully sequenced and contains 1.73 Mbp in length. Chromosome 3 is also fully sequenced and is 2.59 Mpb in length. Finally, chromosome 4, which is the only submetacentric one, it is partially sequenced because it contains an assembly gap that has not been solved and is 2.62 Mbp in length. The structural features of the *B. bovis* genome are similar to those of *Theileria parva* but have major differences with *Plasmodium falciparum* (**Table 1**), despite the fact that *B. bovis* and *P. falciparum* share similar clinical and pathological features [9].

B. bovis contains two extrachromosomal genomes: a lineal mitochondrial genome of 6 Kbp and an apicoplast genome that is circular and consists of 33 kpb with 32 genes and 25 sequences of tRNA.

Features	Species		
	P. falciparum	***T. parva***	***B. bovis***
Size (Mbp)	22.8	8.3	8.2
Number of chromosomes	14	4	4
Total G+C composition (%)	19.4	34.1	41.8
Size of apicoplast genome (kbp)	35	39.5	33
Size of mitochondrial genome (kbp)	~6 linear	~6 linear	~6 linear
Number of nuclear protein coding genes	5,268	4,035	3,671
Average protein coding gene length (bp)[a]	2,283	1,407	1,514
Percent genes with introns	53.9	73.6	61.5
Mean length of intergenic region (bp)	1,694	405	589
G+C composition of intergenic region	13.8	26.2	37
G+C composition of exons (%)	23.7	37.6	44
G+C composition of introns (%)	13.6	25.4	35.9
Percent coding	52.6	68.4	70.2
Gene density[b]	4,338	2,057	2,228

[a]Not including introns.
[b]Genome size/number of protein coding genes.
doi:10.1371/journal.ppat.0030148.t001

Table 1. Genome characteristics of *B. bovis, T. parva* and *P. falciparum* [9].

The apicoplast, which is an organelle conserved in the phylum apicomplexa, is a nonphotosynthetic plastid essential for survival [12]. The apicoplast genome was first sequenced in 1974 from *Plasmodium lophurae* and was thought that it could be mitochondrial DNA. In 1994 it was finally related to plastids DNA when a gen coding for a protein of 470 amino acids in length was identified and it contained a 50% identity with a protein only described in the plastome of red algae [13]. It is believed that the plastid is derived from a secondary endosymbiosis from red algae like in dinoflagellates [14]. Furthermore, *Chromera velia* has a plastid originated from red algae that is closely related with the apicoplast [15].

3. *Babesia* multigenic families

3.1. Variant erythrocyte surface antigen-1

Even though the apicoplast is an apicomplexa organelle, they share a complex of organelles that is characteristic of the apicomplexa: the apical complex. This complex is composed of spherical body, rhoptries and micronemes; in this organelle, different proteins involved in the life cycle are generated, and some of these are secreted to the media or directed to the membrane [16–18]. In the erythrocyte stage, some *Babesia* parasites, including *B. bovis* and *bigemina*, can invade the host erythrocytes in a directly way without a pre-erythrocyte stage. Antigenically, the surface of infected erythrocytes is different between *Babesia* strains and the parasitized erythrocytes present in an infected bovine could fluctuate widely over time, in a process called antigenic variation [19–21]. This process on the infected erythrocytes is carried out by the antigenically variant protein named the variant erythrocyte surface antigen-1 (VESA1) that is constituted by two subunits (a and b) and encoded in a multigene family; the genes *ves-1* involved in this family are related too in cytoadherence and are distributed in the four chromosomes of *Babesia* [19, 22, 23]. Although more of 350 genes *ves-1α* and more of 80 genes *ves-1β* were previously reported, in *B. bovis* genome only 119 were evidenced [9].

3.2. SmORFs

The family of genes *ves-1* is associated across all four chromosomes with another multigene family of proteins that are smaller in size than the *ves-1* genes (**Figure 1**), due to small open reading frames (SmORFs). This family is the second largest in the *B. bovis* genome and comprises 44 genes without significant sequence identity to any protein or gene sequence available in databases. Of 44 genes, 42 are codified in a single exon, but from these 44 proteins that are extracellular just one does not have a signal peptide [9]. Sequence analysis in the T2Bo and Mo7 strains demonstrated that the repertoire varies between strains and has multiple semi-conserved and variable blocks; this family comprises two major branches called SmORFs A and B, and these branches are defined by a large hypervariable insertion in 20 genes [24]. Although the function of these proteins is unknown, it is believed that it could play a functional role in VESA1 biology or contribute to the antigenic variation and immune evasion as a consequence [9, 24].

3.3. VMSA

In American strains, the variable merozoite surface antigen (VMSA) family contains the proteins MSA-1, MSA-2a$_1$, MSA-2a$_2$, MSA-2b and MSA-2c, while in Australian strains only tree genes were found: *msa-1*, *msa-2c* and *msa-2a/b* [25]. The genes that conform this family reside

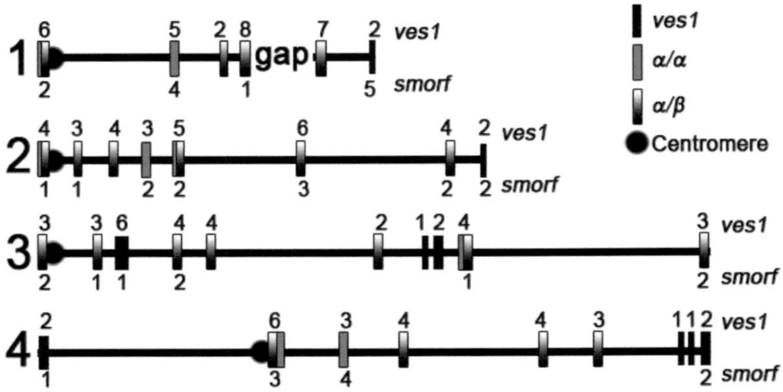

Figure 1. Representation of *B. bovis* chromosomes and the localization of the centromeres, *ves1*, and *smorf* genes. The chromosomes are depicted by black lines, with the chromosome number shown on the left. *ves1* loci are depicted with boxes: Black boxes represent unclassified *ves1* genes; Grey boxes represent at least one *ves1α/ves1α* pair within the cluster; Shaded boxes represent at least one *ves1α/ves1β* pair within the cluster. The number of *ves1* and *smorf* genes is shown above or below each locus, respectively. Finally the centromeres are represented as black circles. Modified from Brayton KA, et al., 2007 [9].

on chromosome 1, and the four copies of *msa2* gene are arranged tandemly in a head-to-tail fashion as long as *msa1* gene is located 5 kbp upstream from the *msa2* genes [9]. These five proteins have a conserved GPI domain and are involved in the first attachment to the erythrocyte. However, the exposed epitopes are not conserved between these proteins of this family and between different strains around the world [18, 26, 27]. Even though these proteins are variable, some studies have been shown that msa-2c gene is the most conserved of this family. Monoclonal antibodies against this protein can recognize strains from different geographic regions, and polyclonal antibodies have an effect on the invasion process, suggesting its utility as recombinant vaccine antigen or in diagnostic tests [18, 26, 28–33]. These results have not been observed in the other MSA proteins; the MSA-1 protein is immunogenic and avoids the invasion process in vitro, but the immunogenic response is not protective [30]. It could be due to the fact that *msa-1* gene has an important allelic variation in strains from the nearby geographical regions. This variation suggests that the antibodies generated could not have a cross-reaction between different strains [34, 35].

3.4. SBP

The spherical body protein (SBP) constitutes another family in *B. bovis*, and these proteins that are located in the spherical body of the apical complex are known as SBP1, SBP2, SBP3 and SBP4. In the invasion process, SBP2 is released from the spherical bodies to the cytoplasmic membrane of the erythrocyte [36]. Twelve truncated copies and just one complete copy of *sbp2* gene were identified, showing a conserved 3′ region in these copies [9, 37]. The complete copy and one truncated are located in the chromosome 4, the other truncated copies are located in the chromosome 3, and some of these truncated copies are expressed in erythrocytic stages of *B. bovis* [10].

3.5. Bbo-6cys

A novel family of genes that codify proteins with similarities to 6cys family of *Plasmodium* were identified in *B. bovis* genome. This family contains six genes (6cys-A, B, C, D, E and F), and these genes are located in tandem in the chromosome 2 except for 6cys-F that is located in a distal region. To identify this family was employed the sequence of the *P. falciparum* PFS230 protein as a query that has a higher homology with Bbo-6cys-E gene. Antibodies against this protein have an inhibitory effect on the invasion process, suggesting its importance in control methods against *B. bovis* infection [38].

3.6. Bovipain

Inhibitors of cysteine proteases have been shown to hamper intraerythrocytic replication of *B. bovis*, and four papain-like cysteine proteases are found in *B. bovis* genome. The bovipain-2, which is the orthologous gene *of P. falciparum* falcipain-2 that is involved in hemoglobin digestion [39], is located in chromosome 4 by an ORF of 1.3 kb without introns, the characterization of this protein shown a molecular weight of 42 kDa, and a transmembrane region and is highly conserved between *B. bovis* strains of North and South America [40]. The bovipain-2 could be employed as a vaccine or as a target of drugs in the babesiosis control.

4. Vaccine antigens

4.1. RON proteins and AMA-1

In *Toxoplasma,* the characterization of the invasion process allowed the identification of a complex of proteins generated in the rhoptry neck, called rhoptry neck proteins (RONs), this family of proteins consists of RON2, RON4, RON5 and RON8 that are related to AMA-1 in the formation of the moving junction (MJ) in the invasion process [41]. The RON complex is inserted into the host cell; meanwhile, AMA-1 is released to the parasite membrane; this process is described in *P. falciparum*, where the specific interaction between the host membrane and the parasite membrane is mediated by AMA-1 and RON2; the disruption of this interaction avoids the invasion process [42, 43]. RON2 was identified in *B. divergens* and *B. microti*, has a full-length sequence of 4053 bp that codifies to a protein of 170 kDa and has apical localization; antibodies against this protein are inhibitors of parasite invasion like in other apicomplexan parasites; The *B. divergens* RON2 protein has a closely related sequence in *B. bovis* identified by BLASTp [42, 44, 45]. The firts protein described to participate in the invasion process as part of the MJ in apicomplexan parasites was AMA-1. This protein is stored in the micronemes and secreted to the apical end during the invasion process. In *Babesia bovis*, AMA-1 contains 606 amino acids and it is codified by a 1818 bp-long gene, without introns. AMA-1 is a type I transmembrane protein with a N-terminal ectodomain, which is divided into three subdomains containing 14 cysteins [18, 46, 47].

4.2. RAP-1

One of the most studied proteins of the rhoptries identified in *B. bovis* is the rhoptry-associated protein 1 (RAP-1). The gene is constituted by only one exon and has a length of 1698 bp with two copies separated by a noncodifying sequence of 1 kbp in *B. bovis* [48]. However in *B. bigemina*, rap-1 is represented by three genes: *rap-1a*, *rap-1b*, and *rap-1c*, arranged in tandem, as explained latter [49]. The members of this family have a signal peptide, four cysteine residues and a 14 aa motive and, moreover, contain immunogenic epitopes B and T that elicit a Th1 humoral response in the host that avoids the attachment of the parasite to the erythrocyte; its structure is conserved between different isolates and is expressed in the sporozoite [37, 50–55].

4.3. MIC

In *B. bovis* was described a gene that codifies to a protein like to the *T. gondii* protein 1 of the micronemes (MIC1). This gene is located in the chromosome 3 and is highly conserved between strains of *B. bovis*. Its function is involved in the cito-adherence process through the binding to sialic acid, and antibodies against the recombinant protein and synthetic peptides designed on antigenic regions of *B. bovis* MIC-1 avoid the invasion process on the in vitro culture of the parasites [56].

4.4. HSP-20

The heat shock protein 20 (HSP-20) is a protein of 20.2 kDa associated with other small proteins related to heat shock in mammals and plants [57]. The *hsp-20* gene consists of 686 bp with an intron of 153 bp that makes a polypeptide of 177 aa [58]. Antibodies against this protein recognize both *B. bovis* and *B. bigemina,* suggesting that HSP-20 contains conserved epitopes in these species [59, 60].

5. *Babesia bigemina*

During the first decade of twenty-first century, the sequencing and description of *B. bovis* genome [61] have helped to find genes that play important roles during its life cycle, currently. The Sanger Institute is leading the sequencing project of *B. bigemina* genome, which is estimated in 10 Mb size distributed in four chromosomes [62]. The advances in genomics of both *Babesia* species that affects cattle in America are allowing researcher to find, analyze, compare and predict proteins involved directly in pathogenesis and its life cycle. For more than five decades, researchers have been trying to develop a vaccine against piroplasmosis; before 1980, several studies were carried out to immunize cattle in an effective way. The first attempts were directed in animals that were infected on purpose and healed from babesiosis as a strategy to avoid nondesirable infections [63]. Some studies were focused on trying to find a way to reduce the virulence of high infective *B. bigemina* strains through inoculum passages in several animals [64], and some even tried to immunize calves in utero [65]. As we know now, the development of a of an effective and low-cost vaccine is more complex than initially thought. Nowadays some countries produce vaccines against bovine babesiosis. The Queensland Government in Australia offers a vaccine made of parasitized bovine blood [66]; this live attenuated parasite vaccine must be stored at −196°C and during its production is necessary a batch of splenectomized calves that must remain in quarantine three times before the first procedures of manufacturing [67]. It is evident that piroplasmosis vaccination involves long periods of production, surgery, and maintenance of animal infected blood donors and thorough procedures to achieve high standards of bioethical considerations.

Currently, research is focused on developing vaccines that avoid complex production procedures and the use of live animals; new technologies have arrived bringing opportunities to develop a vaccine using high throughput production. For this, certain obstacles must be solved before an effective vaccine is produced.

In vaccination, developing gene polymorphisms and antigenic variation is one of the first problems that researchers must cope with, and the selection of most suitable antigen candidates is a crucial step. With gene databases, the analysis of sequence variations has been made easier to find differences in distant geographical strains. In this sense, several studies have been carried out to find whether some proteins are conserved and how auspicious its election as vaccine candidate would be.

Antigenic variation is used by microorganisms as an evasion mechanism of the immune response, and in *Babesia,* the vesa family is the most studied group of genes used to "escape" from the host immune system. As described above for *B. bovis,* the vesa family is composed of two multicopy genes, *ves1α* and *ves1β,* which are distributed within the four chromosomes, and it is estimated that there are 72 and 43 copies of them, respectively. Both genes are located in opposite transcription directions and are governed by a bidirectional promoter followed by small sequences that seem to be incomplete fragments of the same recombined gene. The mechanism proposed for the multiple versions of the protein product of *ves1α* and *ves1β* has to do with the fact that along the genome are *ves* pseudogenes that act like reiterative donors of divergent sequences during several rounds of DNA replications, while the genes that are being transcribed are located in a locus of active transcription, which means that during this multigenic conversion segment event new versions of VESA proteins of *B. bovis* are being generated [68, 69].

Even though in *B. bigemina* antigenic variation as *vesa* family in *B. bovis* is not described, there is information about important genetic differences between strains from diverse geographical locations. On the next lines, we are going to review in general terms some of the genes that are promissory vaccine candidates in *B. bigemina.*

5.1. AMA-1

The apical merozoite antigen (AMA-1) is a protein that has been related to the tight junction complex formation; during this step in the red blood cell invasion, the protein interacts directly with the Rhoptry proteins to anchor both membranes; this process is well studied in the apicomplexan parasite *T. gondii* [70]. In *Babesia* species, AMA-1 as been described as a low-diversity protein; in *B. divergens,* ama-1 was sequenced from nine isolates from France, in which only two punctual mutations were observed compared with the reference strain [71], in *B. bovis,* the analysis of Sri Lankan strains showed that *ama-1* is a conserved member with about 95% of identity; the *msa* genes of this strains were mapped and showed variability. As mentioned previously, *msa* family is highly polymorphic. This last statement proves that the isolates analyzed are different because of their genotype, and among them, there is a highly conserved *ama-1* gene [72]. The *B. bigemina ama-1* seems to be conserved as well, and Italian strains have a conserved sequence among them and considerable differences in comparison with Australian reference strains; however, when these are compared with Mexican and Argentinian reference strains, the sequence matches in a 99% of identity [73]. The conservation level makes AMA-1 an excellent target for vaccine development.

5.2. RAP-1

The Rhoptry Associated Proteins are part of a multigenic family composed in *B. bigemina* of five genes arranged in tandem designated as *rap-1a*; between them, there are two other genes designated as *rap-1b* which is present in the same number of copies as *rap-1a* and at the end of the locus a single copy gene called *rap-1c.* All *rap-1* family members are co-transcribed in merozoites, and some members seem to be conserved in geographical strains [49]. It has been demonstrated in *B. bovis* that specific antibodies are capable of reducing sporozoite invasion to red blood cells in vitro [53]; in *B. bigemina,* antibodies against RAP-1 reduced parasitemia in comparison with an ovalbumin control in calves inoculated with iRBC [74].

5.3. GP45

The product of the *gp45* gene is a glicosylphosphatidylinositol-anchored protein of 45 KDa, which has been related to the adhesion step during the invasion process to red blood cells; it is postulated that play the same role of *msa* family in *B. bovis* [26]. Some studies proved that immunization of calves with the purified GP45 reduced significantly the parasitemia when challenged with a Mexican *B. bigemina* isolate [74]. At this point, GP45 seemed to be an ideal vaccine candidate, however, several years later, other studies demostrated that the gene is not present among all *B. bigemina* strains. Southern Blot analysis revealed that Puerto Rico and St. Croix isolates do not possess *gp45* sequence and also that in Texcoco strain the upstream sequence has polymorphisms and consequently there are nonfunctional promoters. As a result of this, there is a lack of transcription [75]. This last information put in doubt if GP45 would be a good immunological target, not because of its neutralization efficiency but because of that this would not be a good candidate if the purpose of the vaccine is to have a broad-spectrum protection that includes several strains from distant geographical locations.

5.4. Profilin

Profilin is a protein that participates in cytoskeleton ensemble [76]; in *Toxoplasma gondii*, due to its characteristic gliding motility where the cytoskeleton takes part of, profilin has been involved as an important protein to invade host cells and its antigenicity has been proved for its recognition by Toll receptors [77]. There is new evidence that profilin is present in *B. bigemina, B. bovis* and *B. microti,* and more interesting is that sera from infected cattle with *B. bovis* and *B. bigemina* are capable to cross-react with recombinant profilin from both species and even with B. microti; the recombinant cattle babesial profilin is capable of conferring immunity in mice against *B. microti* [78]. Even though there is no information about protective activity in cattle of profilin immunization against *B. bigemina* and *B. bovis,* profilin seems to be another promissory target to work on to achieve an effective vaccine.

The genes mentioned are examples of genes with low variability that can be used as a target to prevent babesiosis by *B. bigemina;* unfortunately, for vaccines developers the variation of sequences and gene products does not follow a high conservation rule. In this sense, experimental strategies have been built up to find a more suitable way to neutralize *Babesia* infection. Taking advantage of the information available on databases and the sequence analysis is possible to track the most appropriate targets. Alignment tools allow researchers to display the protein sequences from several distant geographical strain similarities among their proteins and find the most suitable candidates.

6. New strategies against apicomplexan parasites

There are several studies on *Babesia* proteins, which have an important role on the parasite's life cycle and their immunogenicity. However, even though the protein role on the parasite development has been described in detail, currently there is not a single protein proposed as vaccine candidate against *B. bovis* or *B. bigemina* that generates an immunological protective response as effective as the one produced by the live, attenuated vaccines; the reason of it might be with the fact that one single antigen used as immunogen is not enough to display a strong immunological response. In an attempt to achieve protection against microorganisms, new strategies have been raising and one of them is the design of multiepitopic vaccines; in these novel strategies, *Plasmodium* genus and *Toxoplasma gondii* are some of the microorganisms within the apicomplexan parasites where these methodologies are being applied.

Researchers have been developing vaccines using more than one antigen. Such is the case of *P. falciparum* Chimeric Protein 2.9 (PfCP-2.9) composed of two blood-stage antigens, the carboxyl-terminal region of the protein known as Apical Membrane Merozoite Surface Protein 1 (MSP1–19) and domain III of the Apical Membrane Antigen 1 (AMA-1 III). The PfCP-2.9 resulted in being highly immunogenic in rabbits and in primates and is capable of producing an antibody titer 18-fold higher than both antigens administered in a mixture. The neutralization assays demonstrated that the fusion protein reduces substantially the parasite growth [79].

One concern of last decades is that scientists are predicting that some vector-borne diseases will increase as a consequence of expansion of vector habitats due to global warming [80]. In addition to the fact that vectors are acquiring resistance to pesticides that have been using as a mean of eradication and control, today there are reports that malaria vector exhibits multiresistance to diverse chemical families used for its control leaving any suitable choice to reduce mosquito population [81, 83]. As a novel alternative to cope with this situation, multistage vaccines have been designed in an attempt to interrupt the life cycle in both vertebrate and invertebrate hosts. Using antigens from blood stages as the glutamate-rich protein (GLURP) that had been recognized as a natural antigen in acquiring immunity against malaria [82] and by the usage of sexual stage antigens *Pfp48/45* that are involved in gamete fusion during sexual reproduction within the mosquito vector [83], the central objective of this alternative multiepitope vaccine is to confer immunity in the people that is at risk to acquire the infection and to reduce in long term the infection in the vector avoiding transmission [84]. The usage of more than two antigens is also an opportunity to confer immunity against parasites and to ensure the success to block the infection. In *T. gondii,* an alternative vaccine prototype was designed as a chimeric protein with six predicted epitopes from surface proteins all of them bound in a single polypeptide sequence. This synthetic protein proved to be a good immunogen, and to stimulate CD8+ T cells from seropositive patients in comparison with a mixture of the same antigens and tachyzoite lysates, also the survival percentage in murine models infected with parasites increased substantially in the immunized individuals [85]. The list of new vaccine candidates against *Plasmodium* and *T. gondii* still grows. The information that is generated in these two well-studied models serves as a starting point to extrapolate the strategies and propose new ones in the research of vaccines against apicomplexan parasites. This last section is a very narrow landscape of a long list of options that have been generated against other parasites that for sure are helping scientists to find the effective vaccines against cattle babesiosis.

Author details

Juan Mosqueda[1*], Diego Josimar Hernández-Silva[1,2] and Mario Hidalgo-Ruiz[1,2]

*Address all correspondence to: joel.mosqueda@uaq.mx

1 Laboratory of Immunology and Vaccines, Facultad de Ciencias Naturales, Universidad Autónoma de Querétaro, Querétaro, México

2 Facultad de Ciencias Naturales, Universidad Autónoma de Querétaro, Querétaro, México

References

[1] Tussaint M. Piroplasma bigeminum en Mexico. Bol del Inst Patológico, Estac Agrícola Cent 1. 1905

[2] McCosker PJ. The global importance of babesiosis. In: Babesiosis. Ristic M, Kreier JP, editors. New York: Academic Press; 1981. pp. 1-24

[3] Babes V. Sur l' hémoglobinurie bactérienne du boeuf. Comptes Rendus. Académie des Sciences. 1888;**107**:692-694

[4] Smith T, Kilborne FL. Investigations into the nature, causation, and prevention of Texas or southern cattle fever. Bureau of Animal Industry, Bulletin. 1893;**1**:85-114

[5] Mosqueda J, Falcon A, Ramos JA, Canto GJ, Camacho-Nuez M. Genome and Molecular strategies for Bovine Babesiosis Control. Revista Mexicana de Ciencias Pecuarias. 2012;**3**(Supl 1):51-59

[6] Musoke A, Rowlands J, Nene V, Nyanjui J, Katende J, Spooner P, et al. Subunit vaccine based on the p67 major surface protein of Theileria parva sporozoites reduces severity of infection derived from field tick challenge. Vaccine. 2005;**23**(23):3084-3095

[7] Holec L, Gasior A, Brillowska-Dabrowska A, Kur J. *Toxoplasma gondii*: Enzyme-linked immunosorbent assay using different fragments of recombinant microneme protein 1 (MIC1) for detection of immunoglobulin G antibodies. Experimental Parasitology. 2008;**119**(1):1-6

[8] Ravi G, Ella K, Lakshmi Narasu M. Development of pilot scale production process and characterization of a recombinant multiepitope malarial vaccine candidate FALVAC-1A expressed in *Escherichia coli*. Protein Expression and Purification. 2008;**61**(1):57-64

[9] Brayton KA, Lau AOT, Herndon DR, Hannick L, Kappmeyer LS, Berens SJ, et al. Genome sequence of *Babesia bovis* and comparative analysis of apicomplexan hemoprotozoa. PLoS Pathogens. 2007;**3**(10):1401-1413

[10] de Vries E, Corton C, Harris B, Cornelissen AWCA, Berriman M. Expressed sequence tag (EST) analysis of the erythrocytic stages of *Babesia bovis*. Veterinary Parasitology 2006; **138**(1-2):61–74

[11] Lau AOT, Tibbals DL, McElwain TF. *Babesia bovis*: The development of an expression oligonucleotide microarray. Experimental Parasitology. 2007;**117**(1):93-98

[12] Kohler S, Delwiche CF, Denny PW, Tilney LG, Webster P, Wilson RJ, et al. A plastid of probable green algal origin in apicomplexan parasites. Science. 1997;**275**(5305):1485-1489

[13] Williamson DH, Gardner MJ, Preiser P, Moore DJ, Rangachari K, Wilson RJ. The evolutionary origin of the 35 kb circular DNA of *Plasmodium falciparum*: New evidence supports a possible rhodophyte ancestry. Molecular & General Genetics. 1994;**243**(2):249-252

[14] Zhang Z, Green BR, Cavalier-Smith T. Phylogeny of ultra-rapidly evolving dinoflagellate chloroplast genes: A possible common origin for sporozoan and dinoflagellate plastids. Journal of Molecular Evolution. 2000;**51**(1):26-40

[15] Moore RB, Oborník M, Janouškovec J, Chrudimský T, Vancová M, Green DH, et al. A photosynthetic alveolate closely related to apicomplexan parasites. Nature. 2008;**451**(7181): 959-963

[16] Sam-Yellowe TY. Rhoptry organelles of the apicomplexa: Their role in host cell invasion and intracellular survival. Parasitology Today. 1996;**12**(8):308-316

[17] Preiser P, Kaviratne M, Khan S, Bannister L, Jarra W. The apical organelles of malaria merozoites: Host cell selection, invasion, host immunity and immune evasion. Microbes and Infection. 2000;**2**(12):1461-1477

[18] Yokoyama N, Okamura M, Igarashi I. Erythrocyte invasion by *Babesia* parasites: Current advances in the elucidation of the molecular interactions between the protozoan ligands and host receptors in the invasion stage. Veterinary Parasitology. 2006;**138**(1-2):22-32

[19] Allred DR, Al-Khedery B. Antigenic variation as an exploitable weakness of babesial parasites. Veterinary Parasitology. 2006;**138**(1-2):50-60

[20] Curnow JA. Studies on antigenic changes and strain differences in *Babesia* argentina infections. Australian Veterinary Journal. 1973;**49**(6):279-283

[21] Curnow JA. In vitro agglutination of bovine erythrocytes infected with *Babesia* argentina. Nature. 1968;**217**(5125):267-268

[22] O'Connor RM, Allred DR. Selection of *Babesia bovis*-infected erythrocytes for adhesion to endothelial cells coselects for altered variant erythrocyte surface antigen isoforms. Journal of Immunology (Baltimore, MD 1950). 2000;**164**(4):2037-2045

[23] O'Connor RM, Lane TJ, Stroup SE, Allred DR. Characterization of a variant erythrocyte surface antigen (VESA1) expressed by *Babesia bovis* during antigenic variation. Molecular and Biochemical Parasitology. 1997;**89**(2):259-270

[24] Ferreri LM, Brayton KA, Sondgeroth KS, Lau AOT, Suarez CE, McElwain TF. Expression and strain variation of the novel "small open reading frame" (smorf) multigene family in *Babesia bovis*. International Journal for Parasitology. 2012;**42**(2):131-138

[25] Berens SJ, Brayton KA, Molloy JB, Bock RE, Lew AE, McElwain TF. Merozoite surface antigen 2 proteins of *Babesia bovis* vaccine breakthrough isolates contain a unique hypervariable region composed of degenerate repeats. Infection and Immunity. 2005;**73**(11): 7180-7189

[26] Carcy B, Précigout E, Schetters T, Gorenflot A. Genetic basis for GPI-anchor merozoite surface antigen polymorphism of *Babesia* and resulting antigenic diversity. Veterinary Parasitology. 2006;**138**(1-2):33-49

[27] Lau AOT, Cereceres K, Palmer GH, Fretwell DL, Pedroni MJ, Mosqueda J, et al. Genotypic diversity of merozoite surface antigen 1 of *Babesia bovis* within an endemic population. Molecular and Biochemical Parasitology. 2010;**172**(2-2):107-112

[28] Florin-Christensen M, Suarez CE, Hines SA, Palmer GH, Brown WC, McElwain TF. The *Babesia bovis* merozoite surface antigen 2 locus contains four tandemly arranged and

expressed genes encoding immunologically distinct proteins. Infection and Immunity. 2002;**70**(7):3566-3575

[29] Hines SA, Palmer GH, Jasmer DP, McGuire TC, McElwain TF. Neutralization-sensitive merozoite surface antigens of *Babesia bovis* encoded by members of a polymorphic gene family. Molecular and Biochemical Parasitology. 1992;**55**(1-2):85-94

[30] Hines SA, Palmer GH, Jasmer DP, Goff WL, McElwain TF. Immunization of cattle with recombinant *Babesia bovis* merozoite surface antigen-1. Infection and Immunity. 1995;**63**(1): 349-352

[31] Mosqueda J, McElwain TF, Palmer GH. *Babesia bovis* merozoite surface antigen 2 proteins are expressed on the merozoite and sporozoite surface, and specific antibodies inhibit attachment and invasion of erythrocytes. Infection and Immunity. 2002;**70**(11):6448-6455

[32] Suarez CE, Florin-Christensen M, Hines SA, Palmer GH, Brown WC, McElwain TF. Characterization of allelic variation in the *Babesia bovis* merozoite surface antigen 1 (MSA-1) locus and identification of a cross-reactive inhibition-sensitive MSA-1 epitope. Infection and Immunity. 2000;**68**(12):6865-6870

[33] Wilkowsky SE, Farber M, Echaide I, Torioni de Echaide S, Zamorano PI, Dominguez M, et al. *Babesia bovis* merozoite surface protein-2c (MSA-2c) contains highly immunogenic, conserved B-cell epitopes that elicit neutralization-sensitive antibodies in cattle. Molecular and Biochemical Parasitology. 2003;**127**(2):133-141

[34] Borgonio V, Mosqueda J, Genis AD, Falcon A, Alvarez JA, Camacho M, et al. msa-1 and msa-2c gene analysis and common epitopes assessment in Mexican *Babesia bovis* isolates. Annals of the New York Academy of Sciences. 2008;**1149**:145-148

[35] Leroith T, Brayton KA, Molloy JB, Bock RE, Hines SA, Lew AE, et al. Sequence variation and immunologic cross-reactivity among *Babesia bovis* merozoite surface antigen 1 proteins from vaccine strains and vaccine breakthrough isolates. Infection and Immunity. 2005;**73**(9):5388-5394

[36] Dowling SC, Perryman LE, Jasmer DPA. *Babesia bovis* 225-kilodalton spherical-body protein: Localization to the cytoplasmic face of infected erythrocytes after merozoite invasion. Infection and Immunity. 1996;**64**(7):2618-2626

[37] Dalrymple BP, Peters JM, Goodger BV, Bushell GR, Waltisbuhl DJ, Wright IG. Cloning and characterisation of cDNA clones encoding two *Babesia bovis* proteins with homologous amino- and carboxy-terminal domains. Molecular and Biochemical Parasitology. 1993;**59**(2):181-189

[38] Silva MG, Ueti MW, Norimine J, Florin-Christensen M, Bastos RG, Goff WL, et al. *Babesia bovis* expresses Bbo-6cys-E, a member of a novel gene family that is homologous to the 6-cys family of *Plasmodium*. Parasitology International. 2011;**60**(1):13-18

[39] Shenai BR, Sijwali PS, Singh A, Rosenthal PJ. Characterization of native and recombinant falcipain-2, a principal trophozoite cysteine protease and essential hemoglobinase of *Plasmodium falciparum*. The Journal of Biological Chemistry. 2000;**275**(37):29000-29010

[40] Mesplet M, Echaide I, Dominguez M, Mosqueda JJ, Suarez CE, Schnittger L, et al. Bovipain-2, the falcipain-2 ortholog, is expressed in intraerythrocytic stages of the tick-transmitted hemoparasite *Babesia bovis*. Parasites & Vectors. 2010;**3**:113

[41] Shen B, Sibley LD. The moving junction, a key portal to host cell invasion by apicomplexan parasites. Current Opinion in Microbiology. 2012;**15**(4):449-455

[42] Besteiro S, Michelin A, Poncet J, Dubremetz JF, Lebrun M. Export of a *Toxoplasma gondii* Rhoptry Neck Protein Complex at the Host Cell Membrane to Form the Moving Junction during Invasion. PLOS Pathogens. 2009;**5**(2):1-14

[43] Srinivasan P, Beatty WL, Diouf A, Herrera R, Ambroggio X, Moch JK, et al. Binding of *Plasmodium* merozoite proteins RON2 and AMA1 triggers commitment to invasion. Proceedings of the National Academy of Sciences of the United States of America. 2011; **108**(32):13275-13280

[44] Ord RL, Rodriguez M, Cursino-Santos JR, Hong H, Singh M, Gray J, et al. Identification and characterization of the rhoptry neck protein 2 in *Babesia divergens* and *B. microti*. Infection and Immunity. 2016;**84**(5):1574-1584

[45] Srinivasan P, Ekanem E, Diouf A, Tonkin ML, Miura K, Boulanger MJ, et al. Immunization with a functional protein complex required for erythrocyte invasion protects against lethal malaria. Proceedings of the National Academy of Sciences of the United States of America. 2014;**111**(28):10311-10316

[46] Gaffar FR, Yatsuda AP, Franssen FFJ, de Vries E. Erythrocyte invasion by *Babesia bovis* merozoites is inhibited by polyclonal antisera directed against peptides derived from a homologue of *Plasmodium falciparum* apical membrane antigen 1. Infection and Immunity 2004;**72**(5):2947–2955

[47] Hodder AN, Crewther PE, Matthew ML, Reid GE, Moritz RL, Simpson RJ, et al. The disulfide bond structure of *Plasmodium* apical membrane antigen-1. The Journal of Biological Chemistry. 1996;**271**(46):29446-29452

[48] Suarez CE, Palmer GH, Hötzel I, Hines SA, McElwain TF. Sequence and functional analysis of the intergenic regions separating babesial rhoptry-associated protein-1 (rap-1) genes. Experimental Parasitology. 1998;**90**(2):189-194

[49] Suarez CE, Palmer GH, Florin-Christensen M, Hines SA, Hötzel I, McElwain TF. Organization, transcription, and expression of rhoptry associated protein genes in the *Babesia bigemina* rap-1 locus. Molecular and Biochemical Parasitology. 2003;**127**(2):101-112

[50] Suarez CE, Palmer GH, Jasmer DP, Hines SA, Perryman LE, McElwain TF. Characterization of the gene encoding a 60-kilodalton *Babesia bovis* merozoite protein with conserved and surface exposed epitopes. Molecular and Biochemical Parasitology. 1991;**46**(1):45-52

[51] Suarez CE, McElwain TF, Stephens EB, Mishra VS, Palmer GH. Sequence conservation among merozoite apical complex proteins of *Babesia bovis, Babesia bigemina* and other apicomplexa. Molecular and Biochemical Parasitology. 1991;**49**(2):329-332

[52] Suarez CE, Palmer GH, Hines SA, McElwain TF. Immunogenic B-cell epitopes of *Babesia bovis* rhoptry-associated protein 1 are distinct from sequences conserved between species. Infection and Immunity. 1993;**61**(8):3511-3517

[53] Mosqueda J, McElwain TF, Stiller D, Palmer GH. *Babesia bovis* merozoite surface antigen 1 and rhoptry-associated protein 1 are expressed in sporozoites, and specific antibodies inhibit sporozoite attachment to erythrocytes. Infection and Immunity. 2002;**70**(3):1599-1603

[54] Suarez CE, McElwain TF, Echaide I, Torioni de Echaide S, Palmer GH. Interstrain conservation of babesial RAP-1 surface-exposed B-cell epitopes despite rap-1 genomic polymorphism. Infection and Immunity. 1994;**62**(8):3576-3579

[55] Brown WC, McElwain TF, Ruef BJ, Suarez CE, Shkap V, Chitko-McKown CG, et al. *Babesia bovis* rhoptry-associated protein 1 is immunodominant for T helper cells of immune cattle and contains T-cell epitopes conserved among geographically distant *B. bovis* strains. Infection and Immunity. 1996;**64**(8):3341-3350

[56] Silva MG, Ueti MW, Norimine J, Florin-Christensen M, Bastos RG, Goff WL, et al. *Babesia bovis* expresses a neutralization-sensitive antigen that contains a microneme adhesive repeat (MAR) domain. Parasitology International. 2010;**59**(2):294-297

[57] Lindquist S, Craig EA. The heat-shock proteins. Annual Review of Genetics. 1988;**22**:631-677

[58] Brown WC, Ruef BJ, Norimine J, Kegerreis KA, Suarez CE, Conley PG, et al. A novel 20-kilodalton protein conserved in *Babesia bovis* and *B. bigemina* stimulates memory CD4(+) T lymphocyte responses in *B. bovis*-immune cattle. Molecular and Biochemical Parasitology. 2001;**118**(1):97-109

[59] Montero E, Rodriguez M, Gonzalez L-M, Lobo CA. *Babesia divergens*: Identification and characterization of BdHSP-20, a small heat shock protein. Experimental Parasitology. 2008;**119**(2):238-245

[60] Norimine J, Mosqueda J, Palmer GH, Lewin HA, Brown WC. Conservation of *Babesia bovis* small heat shock protein (Hsp20) among strains and definition of T helper cell epitopes recognized by cattle with diverse major histocompatibility complex class II haplotypes. Infection and Immunity. 2004;**72**(2):1096-1106

[61] Brayton KA, Lau AOT, Herndon DR, Hannick L, Kappmeyer LS, Berens SJ, et al. Genome sequence of *Babesia bovis* and comparative analysis of apicomplexan hemoprotozoa. PLoS Pathogens. 2007;**3**(10):e148

[62] *Babesia bigemina*: Protozoan genomes. The Sanger Institute. [Internet]. 2013. Available from: http://www.sanger.ac.uk/resources/downloads/protozoa/babesia-bigemina.html [Accessed: 2017-03-15]

[63] Mahoney DF, Wright IG, Goodger BV. Immunity in cattle to *Babesia bovis* after single infections with parasites of various origin. Australian Veterinary Journal. 1979;**55**(1):10-12

[64] Dalgliesh RJ, Callow LL, Mellors LT, McGregor W. Development of a highly infective *Babesia bigemina* vaccine of reduced virulence. Australian Veterinary Journal. 1981;**57**(1):8-11

[65] Hall WTK, Tammemagi L, Johnston LAY. Bovine Babesiosis: The immunity of calves to *Babesia bigemina* infection. Australian Veterinary Journal. 1968;**44**(6):259-264

[66] Tick fever vaccines for cattle. The State of Queensland [Internet]. 2015. Available from: https://www.business.qld.gov.au/industries/farms-fishing-forestry/agriculture/livestock/cattle/tick-fever-vaccines [Accessed: 2017-03-15]

[67] Tick fever vaccines for cattle. The State of Queensland [Internet]. 2015. Available from: https://www.business.qld.gov.au/industries/farms-fishing-forestry/agriculture/livestock/cattle/tick-fever-vaccines/vaccine-info [Accessed: 2017-03-15]

[68] Allred DR, Carlton JM-R, Satcher RL, Long JA, Brown WC, Patterson PE, et al. The ves multigene family of *B. bovis* encodes components of rapid antigenic variation at the infected erythrocyte surface. Molecular Cell. 2000;**5**(1):153-162

[69] Al-Khedery B, Allred DR. Antigenic variation in *Babesia bovis* occurs through segmental gene conversion of the ves multigene family, within a bidirectional locus of active transcription. Molecular Microbiology. 2006;**59**(2):402-414

[70] Besteiro S, Michelin A, Poncet J, Dubremetz J-F, Lebrun M. Export of a *Toxoplasma gondii* rhoptry neck protein complex at the host cell membrane to form the moving junction during invasion. PLoS Pathogens. 2009;**5**(2):e1000309

[71] Moreau E, Bonsergent C, Al Dybiat I, Gonzalez LM, Lobo CA, Montero E, et al. *Babesia divergens* apical membrane antigen-1 (BdAMA-1): A poorly polymorphic protein that induces a weak and late immune response. Experimental Parasitology. 2015;**155**:40-45

[72] Sivakumar T, Okubo K, Igarashi I, de Silva WK, Kothalawala H, Silva SSP, et al. Genetic diversity of merozoite surface antigens in *Babesia bovis* detected from Sri Lankan cattle. Infection, Genetics and Evolution 2013;**19**:134-140

[73] Torina A, Agnone A, Sireci G, Mosqueda JJ, Blanda V, Albanese I, et al. Characterization of the apical membrane antigen-1 in Italian strains of *Babesia bigemina*: Characterization of the AMA-1 in *Babesia bigemina*. Transboundary and Emerging Diseases. 2010;**57**(1-2):52-56

[74] McElwain TF, Perryman LE, Musoke AJ, McGuire TC. Molecular characterization and immunogenicity of neutralization-sensitive *Babesia bigemina* merozoite surface proteins. Molecular and Biochemical Parasitology. 1991;**47**(2):213-222

[75] Fisher TG, McElwain TF, Palmer GH. Molecular basis for variable expression of merozoite surface antigen gp45 among American isolates of *Babesia bigemina*. Infection and Immunity. 2001;**69**(6):3782-3790

[76] Schlüter K, Jockusch BM, Rothkegel M. Profilins as regulators of actin dynamics. Biochimica et Biophysica Acta (BBA) – Molecular Cell Research. 1997;**1359**(2):97-109

[77] Plattner F, Yarovinsky F, Romero S, Didry D, Carlier M-F, Sher A, et al. *Toxoplasma* profilin is essential for host cell invasion and TLR11-dependent induction of an interleukin-12 response. Cell Host & Microbe. 2008;**3**(2):77-87

[78] Munkhjargal T, Aboge GO, Ueno A, Aboulaila M, Yokoyama N, Igarashi I. Identification and characterization of profilin antigen among *Babesia* species as a common vaccine candidate against babesiosis. Experimental Parasitology. 2016;**166**:29-36

[79] Pan W, Huang D, Zhang Q, Qu L, Zhang D, Zhang X, et al. Fusion of two malaria vaccine candidate antigens enhances product yield, immunogenicity, and antibody-mediated inhibition of parasite growth in vitro. Journal of Immunology. 2004;**172**(10):6167-6174

[80] Khasnis AA, Nettleman MD. Global warming and infectious disease. Archives of Medical Research. 2005;**36**(6):689-696

[81] Edi CVA, Koudou BG, Jones CM, Weetman D, Ranson H. Multiple-insecticide resistance in Anopheles gambiae mosquitoes, Southern Côte d'Ivoire. Emerging Infectious Diseases. 2012;**18**(9):1508-1511

[82] Soe S, Theisen M, Roussilhon C, Aye K-S, Druilhe P. Association between protection against clinical malaria and antibodies to merozoite surface antigens in an area of hyperendemicity in Myanmar: Complementarity between responses to merozoite surface protein 3 and the 220-kilodalton glutamate-rich protein. Infection and Immunity. 2004;**72** (1):247-252

[83] van Schaijk BCL, van Dijk MR, van de Vegte-Bolmer M, van Gemert G-J, van Dooren MW, Eksi S, et al. Pfs47, paralog of the male fertility factor Pfs48/45, is a female specific surface protein in *Plasmodium falciparum*. Molecular and Biochemical Parasitology 2006; **149**(2):216–222

[84] Theisen M, Roeffen W, Singh SK, Andersen G, Amoah L, van de Vegte-Bolmer M, et al. A multi-stage malaria vaccine candidate targeting both transmission and asexual parasite life-cycle stages. Vaccine 2014;**32**(22):2623-2630

[85] El Bissati K, Chentoufi AA, Krishack PA, Zhou Y, Woods S, Dubey JP, et al. Adjuvanted multi-epitope vaccines protect HLA-A*11:01 transgenic mice against *Toxoplasma gondii*. JCI Insight. 2016;**1**(15):1-18

Chapter 5

Genomics of *Rickettsiaceae*: An Update

Bernardo Sachman-Ruiz and
Rosa Estela Quiroz-Castañeda

Additional information is available at the end of the chapter

http://dx.doi.org/10.5772/intechopen.74563

Abstract

Recent advancements in genomes sequencing of members of *Rickettsiaceae* family have led to set a new landmark in the study of these microorganisms. Genomic analyses of *Rickettsia* and *Orientia* reveal a history of genome reduction because of the interaction with intermediate and final hosts; the evidence shows that this is an ongoing process. The gene loss, the gain, and loss of plasmids in such an easy way, among other significant processes are the evidence of the evolutionary history of this bacterial group involving reductive processes. In particular, the integrative conjugative element called REIS, was necessary in the process of adaption to an intracellular lifestyle in eukaryotes. We present a genomic focusing on *Rickettsia* and *Orientia* species, due to the animal and human importance. In this analysis, the genomic evidence shows that genomes have been extensively shuffled; however the existence of core genes has also been conserved.

Keywords: comparative genomics, *Rickettsia*, pathogens, reductive evolution

1. Introduction

The Rickettsiales are an order within α-proteobacteria that comprises obligate intracellular endosymbionts of arthropods and mammals. Some authors have proposed three pathogenic genera of *Rickettsiales*: (1) *Rickettsiaceae*; (2) *Bartonellaceae*; and (3) *Anaplasmataceae* [1].

More recently, taxonomy of Rickettsiales has changed based on molecular systematics, phylogenomics, and bioinformatics studies. Today, four taxonomic families are recognized: *Anaplasmataceae*, *Rickettsiaceae*, *Ca. Midichloriaceae*, and *Holosporaceae*, with *Rickettsiaceae* being the most well-known group for they are human and animal pathogens [1, 2].

Rickettsiaceae family comprises a large and extremely diverse group of strictly intracellular Gram-negative rod-shaped, non-sporulating, coccoid, and small bacteria. Many of them are obligate intracellular parasites that can infect eukaryotic organisms, including animals and man, through arthropod bites and can cause from mild to severe and even fatal diseases such as epidemic typhus and Rocky Mountain Spotted Fever (RMSF) [1, 3]. This family comprises exclusively two genera: *Rickettsia* and *Orientia*. Both genera contain many known and potential pathogens considered as causative agents of emerging and re-emerging human and animals diseases [1]. Genome size of bacteria of *Rickettsiaceae* are typically small (0.8–2.3 Mbp) mainly due to reductive evolution [4].

These genomes contain split genes, gene remnants, and pseudogenes because of different steps of the genome degradation process. In *Rickettsia*, genomics has revealed extreme genome reduction and massive gene loss compared to less virulent or endosymbiotic species [5].

The *Rickettsiaceae* family has 42 species, 2 belonging to the genus *Orientia* that have been sequenced, and 40 species of the genus *Rickettsia* of which 37 genomes has been sequenced.

This wealth of information reveals a large field of study in comparative genomics to understand the evolution from a free-living to an intracellular or endosymbiotic lifestyle.

Adaptation to intracellular or endosymbiont lifestyle of the family *Rickettsiaceae* is based on the genome degradation process as reducing genes. Additionally, to about 2135 [6] gene remnants and pseudogenes (1622), split genes, and horizontal transfer to other bacterial groups have also been observed. In fact, at least three events in *Orientia* received external genes and *Rickettsia* spp. in six occasions [6].

The generation of *de novo* genes in 17 cases of *Rickettsia* species has been reported, and at least two of them are functional [6]. *Rickettsia* spp. contain gene families, selfish DNA, repeat palindromic elements, genes encoding eukaryotic-like motifs, large fraction of high conserved noncoding DNA, and large fraction of mobile genetic elements (MGEs), including plasmids [5].

The study of the dynamics of genomes evolution of the family *Rickettsiaceae* with regard to new "omics" sciences are driven to understand this extraordinary bacterial group with importance for human and veterinary medicine.

2. Rickettsia

2.1. *Rickettsia* evolution

Apparently, the clade *Rickettsia* diverged from *Claudobacter* 1650-2, 390 million years ago [7]. Then, the primarily lineages infecting arthropods emerged approximately 525–425 million years ago [5, 8]. The emerging of this group has been suggested approximately 150 million years ago after several transitions from a likely free-living ancestor of Rickettsiales to an intracellular life. Nowadays, *Rickettsia* have been discovered in a different hosts as whiteflies, bruchid beetles, ladybird beetles, aphids, among others, which suggest that they are more common than expected [9–12].

http://dx.doi.org/10.5772/intechopen.74563

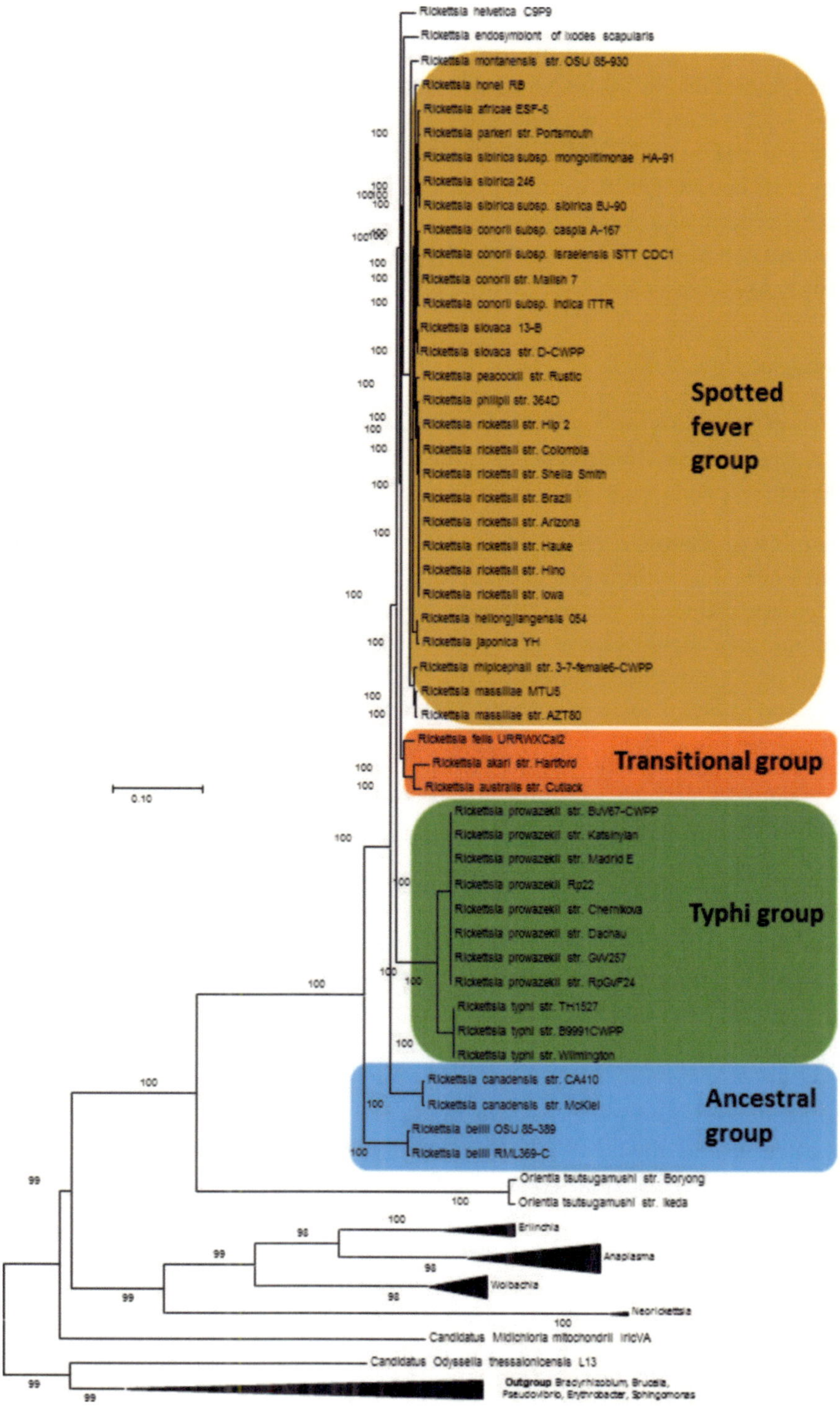

Figure 1. Phylogenetic approximation obtained from amino acid sequences with the online program PATRIC, with the default pipeline (www.patricbrc.org/).

The genus *Rickettsia* comprises pathogenic bacteria causing RMSF, Mediterranean spotted fever, epidemic typhus, and murine typhus [13]. Traditionally, *Rickettsia* was divided into spotted fever and typhus as major groups; however, based on molecular phylogenetic analyses now, it is classified into four groups: (1) ancestral, (2) typhus, (3) transitional, and (4) spotted fever (**Figure 1**). Based on whole genome sequence analysis transitional group was suggested, however, this grouping has generated some controversy based on genetic and genomic criteria and is not widely accepted [5, 14]. The controversy generated by these bacteria classification is because traditional classification methods used in bacteriology are hard to apply to *Rickettsia* spp.

2.2. Genomic of *Rickettsia*

With the use of genome sequence techniques and the characterization of genomic sequences of microorganisms without the need of cultivation, the *Rickettsiaceae* diversity has been explored. Today, 79 genomic sequences of *Rickettsia* and 11 *Orientia* strains are known (**Table 1**).

The availability of complete genome sequences of different *Rickettsia* species led to perform comparative genomic approaches in order to understand bacterial evolution and pathogenesis [5]. Genome reduction is a trait observed in *Rickettsia* species, the gene loss has been an important and ongoing process in evolution of these bacteria. Some intragenus variations in size genome and gene content observed in *Rickettsia* are the consequences of the large diversity of host and infection strategies that these bacteria have developed [5].

The *Rickettsia* genomes exhibit a high degree of synteny punctuated by distinctive chromosome inversions, which goes diminishing as the phylogenetic relationship it is narrower (**Figure 2**).

In general, the genus *Rickettsia* maintains GC content, rRNA, tRNA, and pseudogenes, with only some exceptions (**Table 1**). The aggregate characteristics (number, length, composition, and repeat identity) of tandem repeat sequences of *Rickettsia* which often exhibit recent and rapid divergence between closely related strains and species, are very conserved [15].

2.2.1. Plasmids in Rickettsia

The gene acquisition and gene loss are the major mechanism of adaptation interactions between bacteria and their host, in either the pathogenic or endosymbiotic lifestyle of Rickettsiales and other bacteria. To accomplish this process the preferential vehicle are the plasmids, that encompass very large genetic regions, even more than 100 kilobases (kb) including several set of genes. Their frequent integration at or near tRNA loci suggests that many of them were introduced into bacterial genomes via phage-mediated transfer events. In pathogenicity, they are called "pathogenic islands" and in endosymbionts "symbiotic islands." Recently, the dogma that plasmids are not present in *Rickettsiaceae* was refuted, with the pulsed-field gel electrophoresis (PFGE) and Southern blot analyses of DNAs in different species that suggests that they may be widespread in the genus. Plasmid existence in spite of pressure exerted by reductive genome evolution suggests an important role in rickettsial biology [18].

Taxon_ID	Species	Diseases	Genome _pb	Gene No.	GC	16S_rRNA	23S_rRNA	tRNA	Other RNA	Pseudo_Gene	HGT%
644736402	R_africae	African Tick-Bite Fever	1290917	1077	0.32	1	1	33	0	0	0.56
640753043	R_akari	Rickettsial pox	1231060	1295	0.32	1	1	33	0	0	2.55
2627853922	R_argasii		1437875	1740	0.32	1	1	33	10	0	0.98
2512564059	R_australis		1323280	1297	0.32	1	1	33	0	0	0
2551306119	R_australis		1320572	1556	0.32	1	1	33	5	0	0.58
637000242	R_bellii		1522076	1470	0.32	1	1	34	4	0	0.88
640753044	R_bellii	Epidemic typhus	1528980	1513	0.32	1	1	34	0	0	1.92
2654587808	R_bellii		1543880	1558	0.32	1	1	34	5	0	0.06
2630968994	R_bellii		1618071	1712	0.32	1	1	34	5	0	4.15
640753045	R_canadensis	Epidemic typhus	1159772	1129	0.31	1	1	33	0	0	3.19
2512564031	R_canadensis		1150228	1052	0.31	1	1	33	0	0	0
2548876919	R_conorii	Spotted fever	1249482	1498	0.32	1	1	33	6	0	0.2
637000243	R_conorii	RMSF	1268755	1416	0.32	1	1	33	4	2	0.21
2548877049	R_conorii		1252815	1558	0.32	1	1	33	5	0	0.06
2548877043	R_conorii		1260331	1563	0.33	1	1	33	6	0	0.06
2627853914	R_endosymb._I_pacificus		1564726	1849	0.32	1	1	33	6	0	0.7
647533204	R_endosymb._ I_ scapularis		2100092	2160	0.32	1	1	33	7	0	4.31
2627853651	R_felis		1579101	1775	0.32	1	1	32	5	0	2.65
637000244	R_felis	FbSF, Rickettsiosis	1587240	1552	0.33	1	1	33	4	0	4.45
2648501148	R_felis		1545289	2085	0.32	0	1	33	5	0	0.19
2654587834	R_felis		1485193	1549	0.32	1	1	33	5	0	0
650716082	R_heilongjiangensis		1278471	1333	0.32	1	1	33	0	0	0.08
2597489904	R_helvetica		1417015	1661	0.32	1	1	33	7	0	1.38
2548877054	R_honei		1268758	1510	0.32	1	1	33	5	0	0.07
2630968761	R_hoogstraalii		2303093	2634	0.32	1	1	36	107	0	1.03
2639762805	R_hoogstraalii		1484812	1628	0.32	1	1	33	5	0	0.43
2558860235	R_japonica	Spotted fever	1276675	1439	0.32	1	1	33	5	0	0
2511231062	R_japonica	Spotted fever	1283087	1009	0.32	1	1	33	2	0	0
2627853941	R_massiliae		1266919	1484	0.33	1	1	33	5	0	0.2
641228503	R_massiliae		1376184	1435	0.33	1	1	33	3	416	0.84
2512564029	R_massiliae		1278719	1243	0.33	1	1	33	0	0	0.08
2512564067	R_montanensis		1279798	1253	0.33	1	1	33	0	0	0.08
2512564062	R_parkeri		1300386	1354	0.32	1	1	33	0	0	0.3
2654587812	R_parkeri		1309691	1516	0.32	1	1	34	7	0	0
2654587805	R_parkeri		1300383	1500	0.32	1	1	33	7	0	0
2654587813	R_parkeri		1300534	1504	0.32	1	1	33	7	0	0
644736403	R_peacockii	RMSF, Typhus	1314898	984	0.33	1	1	34	0	0	0.81
2512564043	R_philipii		1287740	1380	0.32	1	1	33	0	0	0.22
2541047049	R_prowazekii		1109301	956	0.29	1	1	33	0	0	0.21
646862338	R_prowazekii	RMSF, Typhus	1111612	990	0.29	1	1	33	2	0	1.01
2512564053	R_prowazekii		1109804	881	0.29	1	1	33	0	0	0.23
2684623071	R_prowazekii		1111769	919	0.29	1	1	33	5	0	0
2512564077	R_prowazekii		1112101	870	0.29	1	1	33	0	0	0.23
2512564080	R_prowazekii		1111445	879	0.29	1	1	33	0	0	0.23
2512564076	R_prowazekii		1111969	865	0.29	1	1	33	0	0	0.23
2541047975	R_prowazekii		1109257	1006	0.29	0	0	33	0	0	0.2
2512564054	R_prowazekii		1111454	880	0.29	1	1	33	0	0	0.23
2541047974	R_prowazekii		1113970	946	0.29	0	0	33	0	0	0.11
637000245	R_prowazekii	RMSF, Typhus	1111523	875	0.29	1	1	33	4	0	0.11
2512564070	R_prowazekii		1109051	875	0.29	1	1	33	0	0	0.23
2554235386	R_prowazekii		1111520	974	0.29	1	1	33	0	0	0.21
2671180980	R_rhipicephali		1448632	1672	0.32	1	1	33	6	0	0.24
2512564064	R_rhipicephali		1305467	1302	0.32	1	1	33	0	0	0
2627854257	R_rickettsii		1269809	1472	0.32	1	1	35	6	0	0
2512564049	R_rickettsii		1270083	1387	0.32	1	1	34	0	0	0.14
641522647	R_rickettsii	RMSF	1268175	1421	0.32	1	1	34	0	0	0.77
2512564034	R_rickettsii		1255681	1369	0.32	1	1	34	0	0	0.15
2512564047	R_rickettsii		1270751	1345	0.32	1	1	34	0	0	0.07
2512564048	R_rickettsii		1286792	1388	0.33	1	1	37	0	0	0.79
640753046	R_rickettsii	RMSF	1257710	1382	0.32	1	1	34	0	0	0.65
2512564040	R_rickettsii		1269774	1377	0.32	1	1	34	0	0	0.07
2512564030	R_rickettsii		1267197	1380	0.32	1	1	34	0	0	0.14
2627853817	R_rickettsii		1257005	1453	0.32	1	1	34	6	0	0.07
2548876780	R_sibirica	RMSF, Typhus	1254734	1474	0.32	1	1	33	5	0	0.2
2548876922	R_sibirica		1252337	1519	0.32	1	1	33	5	0	0.07
638341178	R_sibirica	North Asian tick typhus	1250021	1270	0.32	1	1	33	0	0	0.08
2512564061	R_slovaca		1275720	1383	0.33	1	1	33	0	0	0.07
2511231061	R_slovaca	Headache, Malaise	1275089	1322	0.33	1	1	33	2	172	0
2582581025	R_sp. ISO7		1657692	1710	0.32	1	1	33	1	31	1.17
2551306549	R_sp. MEAM1		1105028	1395	0.32	3	4	31	5	0	5.88
2518645505	R_sp. PRT001		1317139	1541	0.31	0	3	13	13	0	51.2
2513020046	R_sp. PRT001		934551	1079	0.29	0	0	12	0	0	61.54
2617271228	R_tamurae		1453216	1670	0.32	1	1	33	10	0	0.78
637000246	R_typhi	Typhus	1111496	920	0.29	1	1	33	4	42	2.61
2512564075	R_typhi		1112957	875	0.29	1	1	33	0	0	0.23
2512564057	R_typhi	Typhus	1112372	874	0.29	1	1	33	0	0	0.34
2585427698	R_bacterium Os18		1469252	1485	0.29	1	1	38	3	0	7.21
2599185121	R_ bacterium Ac37b		1917613	1886	0.31	1	1	38	3	0	34.73
2630968804	R_bacterium SCGCAAA041		822563	896	0.33	1	0	13	2	0	21.76
2645727592	Orientia chuto		1092196	1124	0.29	1	1	33	3	0	1.07
2627853971	Orientia tsutsugamushi		1997698	3013	0.3	1	1	28	24	0	0.23
640427127	Orientia tsutsugamushi	Scrub typhus	2127051	2180	0.31	1	1	35	1	959	2.66
2648501828	Orientia tsutsugamushi		2221260	2867	0.3	1	1	34	32	0	0.24
642555145	Orientia tsutsugamushi	Scrub typhus	2008987	2004	0.31	1	1	34	0	0	1.85
2627853710	Orientia tsutsugamushi		1689193	2232	0.31	0	1	28	30	0	1.08
2627853684	Orientia tsutsugamushi		2460104	3094	0.31	1	1	35	39	0	0.26
2639762819	Orientia tsutsugamushi		3033399	4269	0.3	2	1	57	30	0	0.19
2627853773	Orientia tsutsugamushi		712858	942	0.3	1	0	10	7	0	0.11
2645727557	Orientia tsutsugamushi		1478442	1643	0.3	1	1	35	35	0	0.61
2627854151	Orientia tsutsugamushi		1454354	1624	0.3	1	1	34	22	0	0.43
RMSF = Rocky Mountain Spotted Fever		**FbSF = Flea-borne Spotted Fever**									

Table 1. *Rickettsiaceae* family genomes data reported on img.jgi.doe.gov.

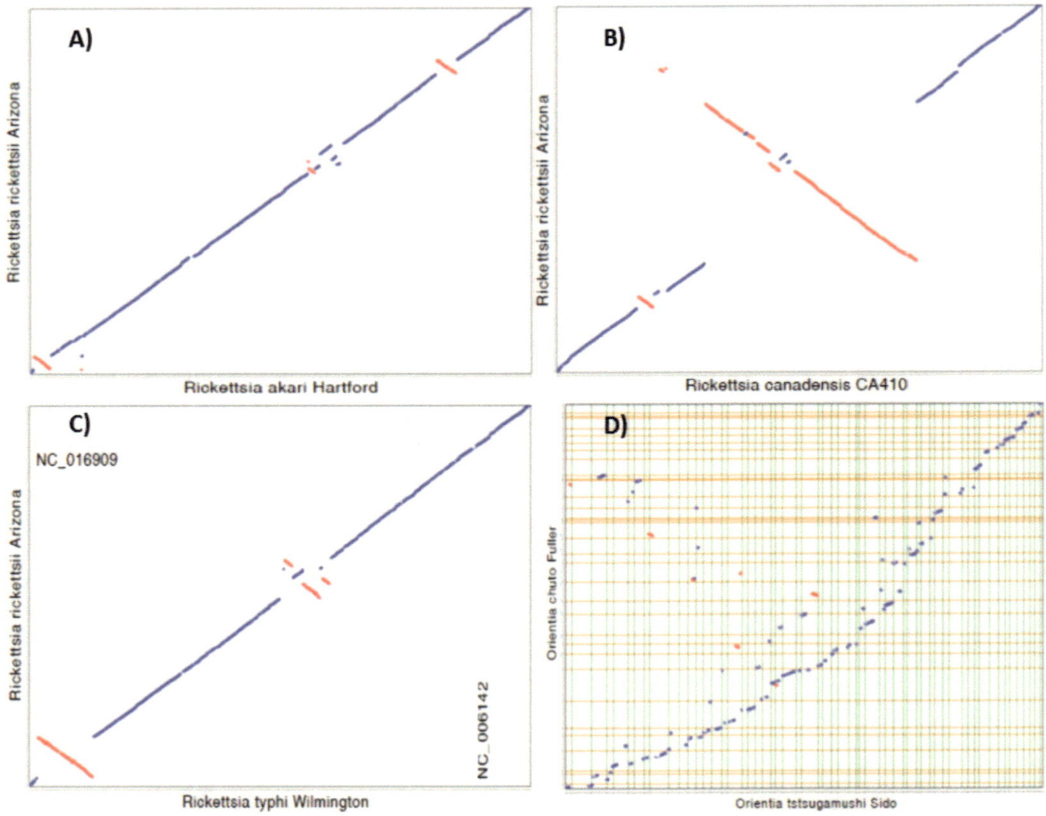

Figure 2. Comparison of pairwise syntenic dot plots of the nucleotide sequences: (A) *Rickettsia rickettsii* Arizona vs. *R. akari*; (B) *R. rickettsii* vs. *R. canadensis* CA410; (C) *R. rickettsii* vs. *R. typhi* Wilmington; and (D) *Orientia chuto* Fuller vs. *O. tsutsugamushi* Sido.

In the most relevant study of plasmids in *Rickettsia* with 26 species, the authors found that 11 species had 1 to 4 plasmid(s) with a size ranging from 12 to 83 kb, and contained 15 to 85 genes. They elucidated that pRICO, the last common ancestor of the current rickettsial plasmids, was vertically inherited mainly from *Rickettsia*/*Orientia* chromosomes and diverged vertically into a single or multiple plasmid(s) in the species [3].

Out of 747 protein-coding genes, 65% were full-length genes and 35% were partially degraded. Degradation levels varied among plasmids, ranging from 16 to 40% in larger plasmids (size >47 kbp) and 44 to 59% in smaller plasmids [3].

It has been observed that plasmids are lost during long-term serial passage in cultured cells, which complicate studies of ancestry to elucidate a single or multiple ancestors. Nevertheless plasmids clustered into four putative groups (I–IV) (**Figure 3**): group I included four large and three small plasmids of five species: pRra2 in *R. raoultii*, pRhe in *R. helvetica*, pRfe, pRfel1, and pdRfe in *R. felis*, pRam32 in Candidatus *R. amblyomii*, and pRau in *R. rhipicephalii*; group II clustered two large and four small plasmids belonging to five species: pReis1 and pReis2 in *R.* endosymbiont of *Ixodes*, pRaf in *R. africae*, pRam23 in C. *R. amblyomii*, pRmo in *R. monacensis*, and pRpe in *R. peacokii*; group III contain five small plasmids of four species:

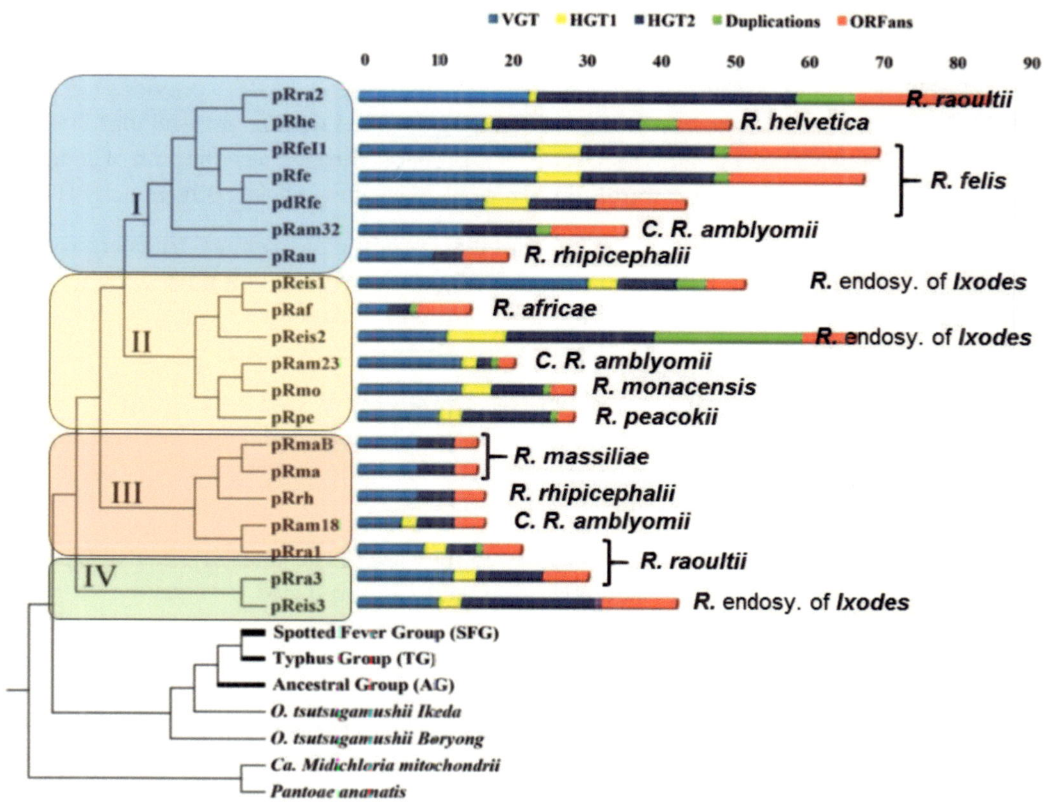

Figure 3. Evolutionary events that shaped rickettsial plasmids. Plasmid supertree obtained from 10 genes of *Rickettsia* and *Orientia* species. The genes used were hsp, dnaA, sca12, transposase 1 and 2, phospholipase, traD, leucine repeat, helix-turn-helix, and thymidylate kinase. Figure based on [3].

pRam18 in C. *R. amblyomii*, pRrh in *R. rhipicephalii*, pRra1 in *R. raoultii* and pRma and pRmaB in *R. massiliae*; and group IV gathered one large and one small plasmids from two species: pReis3 in *R.* endosymbiont of Ixodes and pRra3 in *R. raoultii*. At inter-species level, plasmids of the same group showed variable sequence conservations [6].

Rickettsia plasmids are a mirror of the evolutionary history of this bacterial group involving reductive processes, duplication events, and horizontal acquisition of genes necessary to adapt to an intracellular lifestyle in eukaryotes. It is now necessary to determine their distribution, evolution, and their role in host adaptation and virulence [16].

2.2.2. *Gene loss and evolution of Rickettsia*

The mechanism of gene loss it has been a fairly widespread strategy in the evolution of the Rickettsiales genomes, and was discovered in the *Rickettsia* endosymbiont *Ixodes scapularis* (REIS). It was found that proliferation of mobile genetic elements, in particular, an integrative conjugative element RAGE (for Rickettsiales Amplified Genetic Element) is present in chromosome and plasmids [6].

REIS encodes nine conserved RAGEs that include F-like type IV secretion systems similar to other in *Rickettsia* genomes. These comprise 35% of the total genome, making REIS one of the most plastic and repetitive bacterial mobile elements. The presence of REIS provides the most convincing evidence that conserved rickettsial genes associated with an intracellular lifestyle were acquired via MGEs, especially the RAGE. This, probably through a continuum of genomic invasions, provides insights about the origin of mechanisms of rickettsial pathogenicity [17].

The RAGEs are the fusion of *tra*-like family genes that encoding the conjugal transfer protein. Inserted genes can be found between *traA* and *traD* genes. We present a phylogeny with 60 sequences of *traD* genes of 16 genomes species (**Figure 4**), including ancestral, transitional, and spotted fever group.

Rickettsia spp. share 1027 genes that probably were vertically transferred from "proto-*Rickettsia*" *R. bellii* maintained all these genes and other species lost a large part of them, like *R. prowazekii* and *R. typhi* (128 lost genes). It is well supported that differential gene loss contributes to creation of new rickettsial species [6].

In conclusion, the loss of regulatory genes causes an increase of virulence in rickettsial species in ticks and mammals, and the *tra* operon is presumably involved [18].

2.2.3. Phylogeny and taxonomy of Rickettsia

The taxonomy of *Rickettsia* was historically based on the phenotypic criteria, the phylogenetic approaches with gene 16S rRNA defined three groups typhus group (TG) which includes: *R. prowazekii* and *R. typhi*; classic spotted fever group (SFG), which includes a large collection of mostly tick-borne rickettsials; and an ancestral group (AG), which included *R. bellii* and *R. canadensis* [19], even thus they remain unresolved clades at species level.

Other evolutionary gen reconstructions are inconsistent when using different portions of the genome [20]. An analysis based on the whole genome sequence analysis (WGSA) allows emerging of transitional group (TRG) consisting of *Rickettsia felis* which was primarily associated with *Ctenocephalides felis* and the sister group to the neighboring: *R. akari* [19, 20].

In different studies of *Rickettsia* using WGSA, we can observe resolved trees with single topology, which is supported by multiple sources of phylogenetic signal, which describes the evolutionary history of the core genome [20].

Unfortunately, we cannot have always the powerful tool of WGSA, so the search of new molecular markers is necessary to provide a well-supported phylogenetic approach, at least at species level. As we can see in **Figure 5**, a reliable phylogeny can be obtained using several sequences of all *Rickettsia* species and the conserved gen *rpoB*, offering high-resolution clades at species level.

2.2.4. Comparative genomics of Rickettsia

In the existing 82 sequenced genomes of *Rickettsia* species, 77 belong to 37 species and 5 in *Candidatus* status. In general, the genomes size is constant, between 0.8 and 2.3 Gb; and the average size is 1.3 Gb.

The genomes shows 865 genes as minimum and a maximum of 2634 genes, the average is 1360 genes; the GC content is very constant among genomes with 33%. Only four genomes have

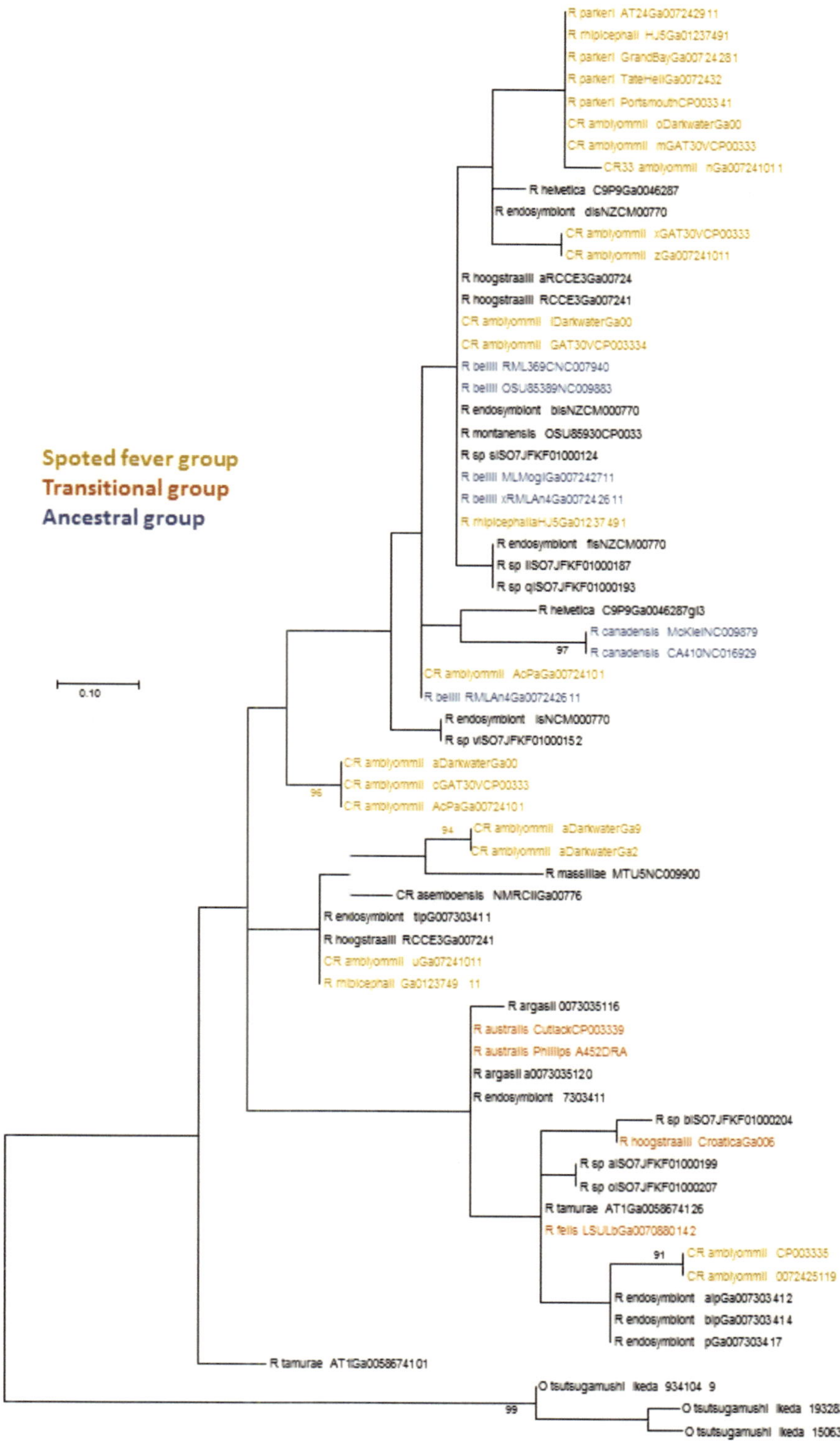

Figure 4. The evolutionary history of gen TraD was inferred by using MEGA7 using ML method and GTR model, with the highest log likelihood (−237.1216). The analysis involved 60 nucleotide sequences from genomes of the IMG (img.jgi.doe.gov) of 16 species and tree outgroup from NCBI.

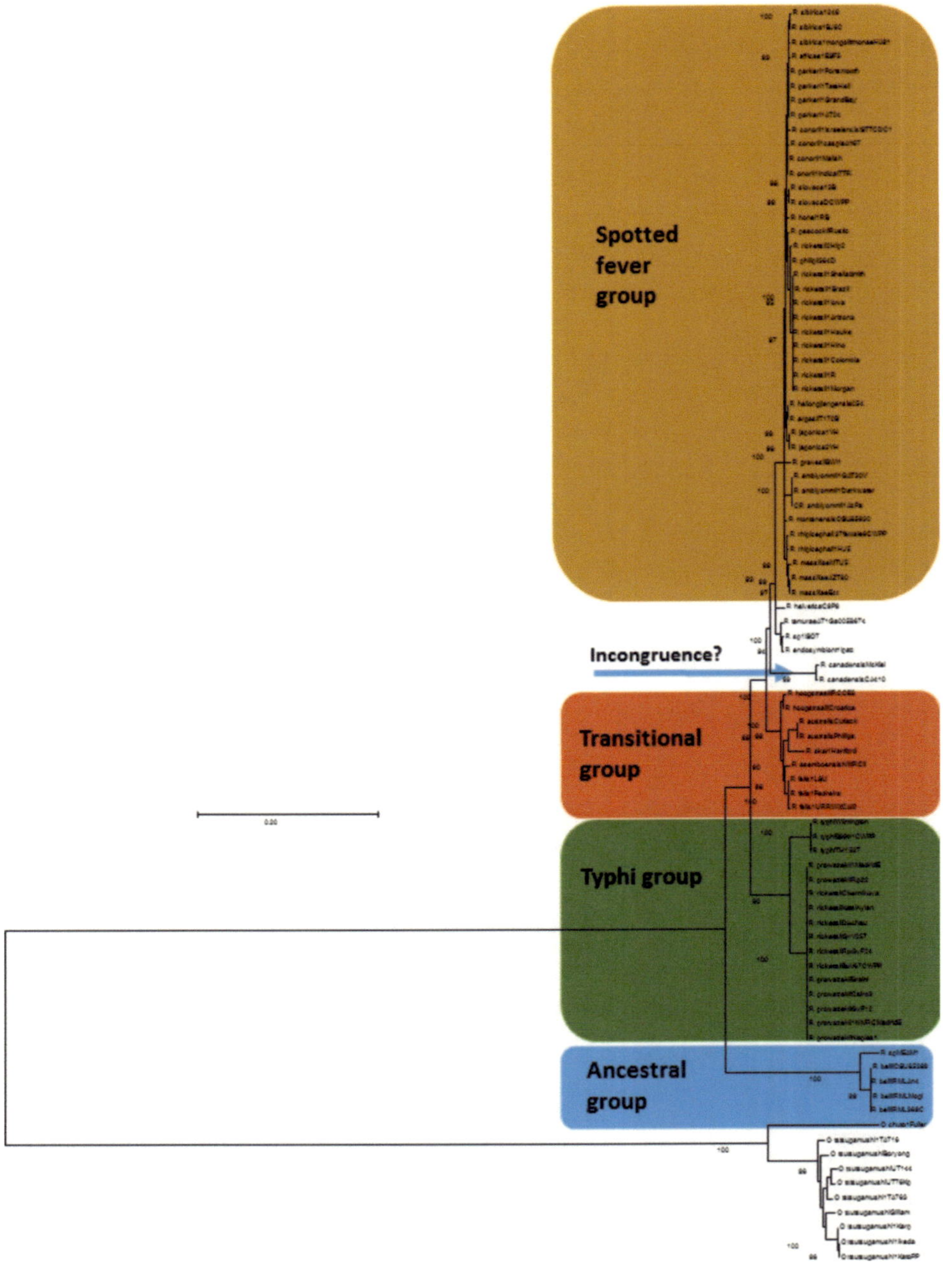

Figure 5. *rpoB* Phylogeny of *Rickettsia* and *Orientia* was inferred by using MEGA7 using ML method and GTR model, with the highest log likelihood (−14425.5668). The analysis involved 87 nucleotide sequences obtained from genomes of the IMG site img.jgi.doe.gov. There were a total of 2721 positions in the final dataset.

pseudogenes and the average of horizontal gene transfer is 2.87% (**Table 1**). The presence of conjugative elements in some of these genomes correlates with an increased number of transposons, breakpoints, and a general breakdown in genome synteny, which is very conserved

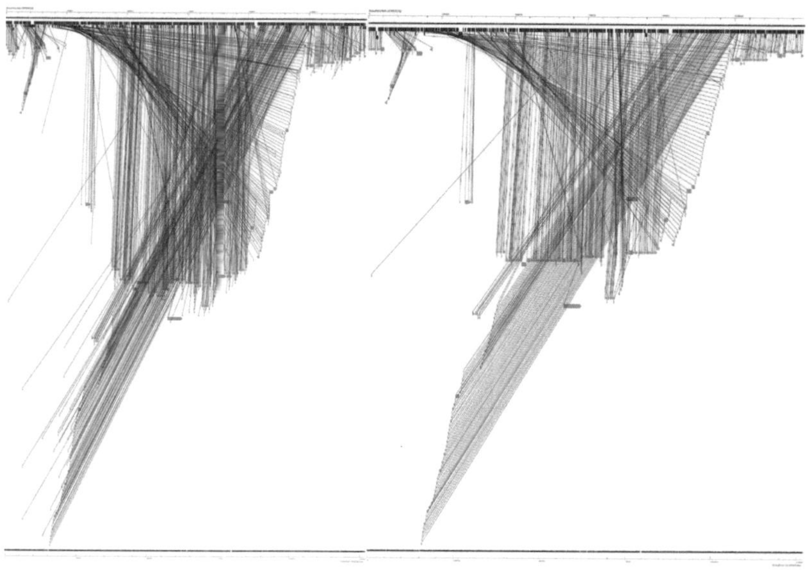

Figure 6. Genomic rearrangements with different cutoff: (A) 100 bp; (B) 1000 pb.

in nearby groups, with some inversions. However, as they move away phylogenetically, more inversions are observed and still synteny is conserved (**Figure 2**).

The genomic and metabolic impairment of *Rickettsia* genomes is mainly due to population bottlenecks in free live style and genome size reduction is related to the gene loss, split genes, and pseudogene formation during endosymbiosis. The presence of plasmids and their sporadically integration into the chromosome leading to emergence of pathogenicity and loss of regulation are also factors that influence in *Rickettsia* genomes variability [5].

When comparing synteny between *Rickettsia rickettsii,* member of spotted fever group, and *R. felis*, member of transitional group, (**Figure 6**) a panoramic view of the genome dynamics at large scale can be observed. A point cut of 100 pb events shows a significant difference respect to 1000 pb. This difference is also observed in the gen itself and the alignment with the Vista tool in the IMG site (img.jgi.doe.gov/cgi-bin/w/main.cgi?section=Vista&page=vista).

The comparative genomic studies reveal the relation between small size and more virulent species strains, this fact supports *Rickettsia* virulence and is the result of a reduction genome ongoing process. The reconstructions of inactive genes revealed that deletions strongly predominate over insertions with an excess of GC-to-AT substitutions, which explain the low GC content (32% in genome average) [21].

3. *Orientia*

This genus comprises *Orientia tsutsugamushi*, the causative agent of scrub typhus or Tsutsugamushi disease, and the novel species *Orientia chuto* identified in Dubai, in the United

Arab Emirates [22, 23]. Humans are the final host of the bacteria and the symptoms include a simple febrile illness to a life threatening fatal infection (meningitis, eschar, disseminated intravascular coagulation) and complicated with dysfunction in several organs [24].

O. tsutsugamushi is widely spread in the Asia-Pacific region comprising Siberia, Japan, Korea, Papua New Guinea, Thailand, Philippines, the Kamchatka Peninsula in the east, Pakistan in the west, and down to Australia in the south [22, 25].

These bacteria are an obligate intracellular Gram-negative rod-shaped and its vector is *Leptotrombidium* spp. species mite populations, where vertically is maintained. Transmission to humans occurs by the bite of infected larval-stages mites called chiggers [26]. Although, some other vectors have been reported, including ticks of rodents from different geographic origins [27, 28]. Vertical or transovarial transmission of *Orientia* spp. would be essential to the maintenance of the infection due to mites have a role as vectors and reservoir [25].

In the recent years, a dramatic variation in phenotypes and genotypes of *O. tsutsugamushi* has been observed in humans, animal host, and vector mites using immunological and molecular methods [25].

3.1. Genotyping of *Orientia*

Strain classification of *Orientia* and serotyping were performed based on the immunodominant 56 kDa type-specific antigen (TSA) located on the surface of the bacteria [29].

With this method, three antigenic prototypes were primarily described: Karp, Kato, and Gilliam; and then many more variations of different serotypes were described in several countries [30, 31]. As primary attempts, genotyping was made by sing RFLP (Restriction Fragment Length Polymorphism) to identify unique isolates or directly by sequence analysis of the TSA gene by PCR. A comparison between nested polymerase chain reaction (nPCR) of 56-kDa antigen gene, the most used molecular technique for confirmation of scrub typhus and genotyping of *O. tsutsugamushi,* and single-step conventional PCR (cPCR) revealed that nPCR products have more variation among strains than cPCR, which emphasizes cPCR advantages [32, 33].

The antigenic variation of the strains Karp, Kato, and Gilliam, subsequent strains, and recently isolates discovered depends on the diversity of the TSA located on the surface of *O. tsutsugamushi [34].*

Genome of *O. tsutsugamushi* strain Boryong has 2,217,051 bp, with 2179 potential protein-coding sequences and 963 sequences of fragmented genes, which represent a coding capacity of only 49.6%. A core genome is composed of 512 genes that share with seven *Rickettsia* species (**Figure 7**). The fragmented regions have a significant interest since they correspond to repeated DNA regions distributed throughout the whole genome. The absent of collinearity with other *Rickettsia* genomes and the no systematic pattern in the GC plot suggest that the genome has been extensively shuffled [35].

3.2. Comparative genomics

Nakayama et al. [36] compared two genomes of *O. tsutsugamushi*: Boryong and Ikeda strains. Both genomes recently reported and isolated in Korea and Japan [35, 37]. In this

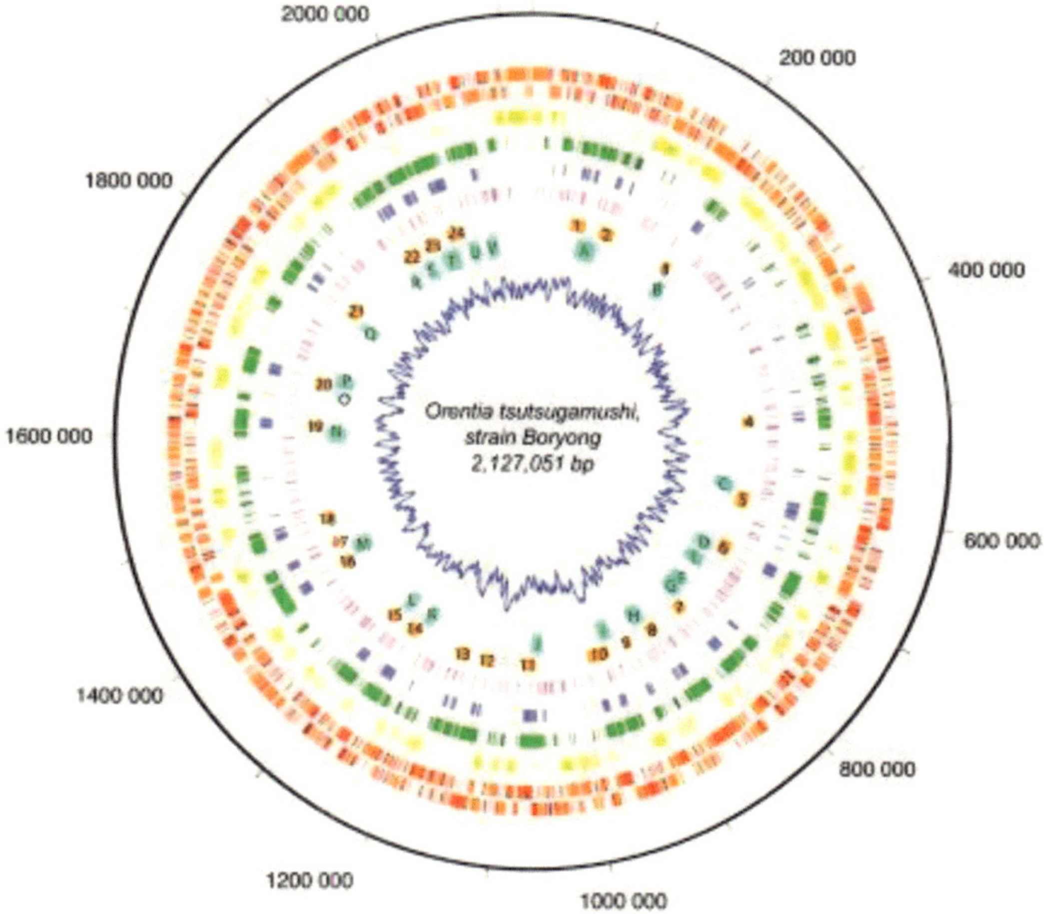

Figure 7. The mapping of different regions in the circular genome of *O. tsutsugamushi*. Figure reproduced from [35].

comparative analysis, a phylogenetic relationship of *O. tsutsugamushi strains* was reconstructed using 11 conserved genes in *O. tsutsugamushi* and closely related *Rickettsia* species. The multilocus sequencing analysis of 10 *O. tsutsugamushi* strains representing each TSA subtype revealed the distribution of strain-specific sequences identified in Boryong or Ikeda among the *O. tsutsugamushi* strains.

The analysis revealed an extensive reductive genome evolution and a significant amplification of repetitive sequences. In fact, the repetitive sequences identified in Ikeda strain were classified in three types: (1) Integrative and conjugative element (ICE) named OT amplified genetic element (OtAGE); (2) Transposable elements (TE); and (3) Short repetitive sequences of unknown origin (short repeat). Both genomes of *Orientia* contain the same set of repetitive sequences, which have been amplified in both strains and caused an extensive genome shuffling. Additional to this, the existence of core genes set of family Rickettsiaceae is also highly conserved. It seems that the extensive genome rearrangements generated by repetitive sequences have occurred between the two strains, although the high complex and repeat-rich feature of the *Orientia* genomes and some genomics differences still have to be clarified [36].

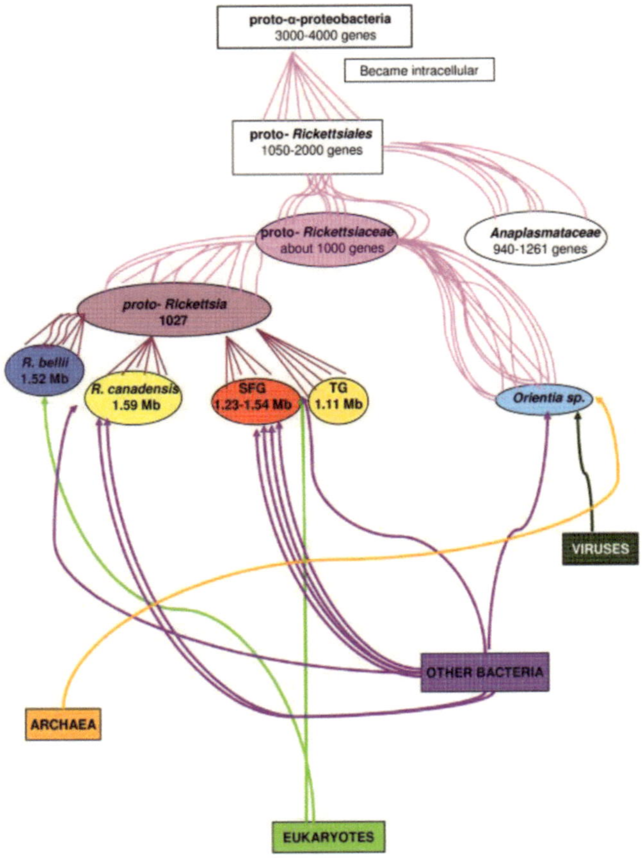

Figure 8. Probable gene gain events occurred in *Rickettsia* and *Orientia*. *Orientia* would have been gained genes from viruses, other bacteria and even archaea. Figure taken from [38].

3.3. Gene loss, gene gain, and evolution

Reductive evolution can be studied in members of *Rickettsiales*, because genome degradation is a process that occurs in members of this order. Gene loss has shaped the content of some *Rickettsiales* genomes, and horizontal gene transfer (HGT) has played an important role in the genome evolution of these bacteria [38].

An evolution study based on gene loss and HGT events in *Rickettsia* spp., *Anaplasma* spp. and *Orientia* spp. showed that three possible HGT event occurred from various organisms to *Orientia* and six events to *Rickettsia* spp., and three possible HGT event from *Rickettsia* and *Orientia* to other bacteria (**Figure 8**) [38].

Gene gain is a known event that has occurred throughout rickettsial evolution. In *O. tsutsugamushi* Ikeda one HGT event was identified and none in *O. tsutsugamushi* Boyrong. Many of the genes transferred by HGT were gained ancestrally, and include transposases and ankyrin repeat-containing proteins that appear to have been transferred from viruses and protist to *Orientia* species; the genes donated by *Orientia* were gained by *Firmicutes* spp., *Bacteroidetes* spp., and *Gamma-proteobacteria* spp. [38].

The whole genome analysis of *O. tsutsugamushi* Boryong has revealed the presence of type IV secretion system histidine kinases, SpoT, Tra, and ankyrin repeat- and tetratricopeptide repeat (TPR) containing proteins. Histidine kinases are proteins that act as sensor and signal transduction in response to changes in the environment; SpoT family proteins have a role in the response to energy starvation; Tra family proteins participate in gene transfer between rickettsia and other bacteria [39].

In a shotgun proteomics analysis using SDS-PAGE and LC-MSMS, many expressed proteins and the protein profiles were identified. 584 out of 1152 proteins of *O. tsutsugamushi* were identified by trypsin and Lys-C digestion and LC-MSMS, which corresponds to 49.4% proteins, annotated on the genome of the bacteria. It seems that during evolution the obligate intracellular bacteria lacked some proteins of important function (i.e., metabolism) and conserved proteins that allow them to survive in the host cells [39].

4. Conclusions

Rickettsiaceae family comprises widely distributed and genomically diverse microorganisms. Genome analysis of the members of the family has revealed an extraordinary evolution process throughout the time driven by the constant interactions with host cells and other bacteria. Recently, genomics analyses have revealed the presence of core genes in this family, as well as genes encoding proteins with significant function in *Orientia* spp.

Author details

Bernardo Sachman-Ruiz* and Rosa Estela Quiroz-Castañeda

*Address all correspondence to: sachman.bernardo@inifap.gob.mx

Anaplasmosis Unit, National Center for Disciplinary Research in Veterinary Parasitology, CENID-PAVET, INIFAP, Jiutepec, Morelos, México

References

[1] Gillespie J, Beier-Sexton M, Azad A. The Family Rickettsiaceae. In: Practical Handbook of Microbiology. Second Ed. [Internet] ed. Boca Raton, USA: CRC Press; 2008;(April 2015). pp. 445-456. Available from: http://www.crcnetbase.com/doi/abs/10.1201/9781420009330.ch28

[2] Martijn J, Schulz F, Zaremba-Niedzwiedzka K, Viklund J, Stepanauskas R, Andersson SGE, et al. Single-cell genomics of a rare environmental alphaproteobacterium provides unique insights into *Rickettsiaceae* evolution. The ISME Journal. 2015:1-13

[3] El Karkouri K, Pontarotti P, Raoult D, Fournier PE. Origin and evolution of rickettsial plasmids. PLoS One. 2016;**11**(2):1-17

[4] Darby AC, Cho N-H, Fuxelius H-H, Westberg J, Andersson SGE. Intracellular pathogens go extreme: Genome evolution in the *Rickettsiales*. Trends in Genetics. 2007;**23**(10):511-520

[5] Merhej V, Raoult D. Rickettsial evolution in the light of comparative genomics. Biological Reviews. 2011;**86**(2):379-405

[6] Georgiades K, Merhej V, El Karkouri K, Raoult D, Pontarotti P. Gene gain and loss events in *Rickettsia* and *Orientia* species. Biology Direct [Internet]. 2011;**6**(1):6. Available from: http://www.biology-direct.com/content/6/1/6

[7] Battistuzzi FU, Feijao A, Hedges SB. A genomic timescale of prokaryote evolution: insights into the origin of methanogenesis, phototrophy, and the colonization of land. BMC Evolutionary Biology [Internet]. 2004;**4**(1):44. Available from: http://www.biomedcentral.com/1471-2148/4/44

[8] Weinert LA, Werren JH, Aebi A, Stone GN, Jiggins FM. Evolution and diversity of *Rickettsia* bacteria. BMC Biology. 2009;**7**:6

[9] Gottlieb Y, Ghanim M, Chiel E, Gerling D, Portnoy V, Steinberg S, et al. Identification and localization of a *Rickettsia* sp. in *Bemisia tabaci* (Homoptera: Aleyrodidae). Applied and Environmental Microbiology. 2006;**72**(5):3646-3652

[10] Fukatsu T, Shimada M. Molecular characterization of Rickettsia sp. in a bruchid beetle, *Kytorhinus sharpianus* (Coleoptera: Bruchidae). Applied Entomology and Zoology. 1999;**34**(3):391-397

[11] Weinert LA, Tinsley MC, Temperley M, Jiggins FM. Are we underestimating the diversity and incidence of insect bacterial symbionts? A case study in ladybird beetles. Biology Letters. 2007;**3**(6):678-681

[12] Sakurai M, Koga R, Tsuchida T, Meng X-Y, Fukatsu T. Rickettsia symbiont in the pea aphid *Acyrthosiphon pisum*: Novel cellular tropism, effect on host fitness, and interaction with the essential symbiont *Buchnera*. Applied and Environmental Microbiology. 2005;**71**(7):4069-4075

[13] Schroeder CLC, Narra HP, Rojas M, Sahni A, Patel J, Khanipov K, et al. Bacterial small RNAs in the genus *Rickettsia*. BMC Genomics. 2015;**16**:1075

[14] Gillespie JJ, Beier MS, Rahman MS, Ammerman NC, Shallom JM, Purkayastha A, et al. Plasmids and rickettsial evolution: Insight from *Rickettsia felis*. PLoS One. 2007;**2**(3):e266

[15] Eremeeva ME, Madan A, Shaw CD, Tang K, Dasch GA. New perspectives on rickettsial evolution from new genome sequences of rickettsia, particularly *R. canadensis*, and *Orientia tsutsugamushi*. Annals of the New York Academy of Sciences. 2005;**1063**(August 2016):47-63

[16] Baldridge GD, Burkhardt NY, Felsheim RF, Kurtti TJ, Munderloh UG. Plasmids of the pRM/pRF family occur in diverse *Rickettsia* species. Applied and Environmental Microbiology. 2008;**74**(3):645-652

[17] Gillespie JJ, Joardar V, Williams KP, Driscoll T, Hostetler JB, Nordberg E, et al. A rickettsia genome overrun by mobile genetic elements provides insight into the acquisition of genes characteristic of an obligate intracellular lifestyle. Journal of Bacteriology. 2012;**194**(2):376-394

[18] Fournier P-E, El Karkouri K, Leroy Q, Robert C, Giumelli B, Renesto P, et al. Analysis of the *Rickettsia africae* genome reveals that virulence acquisition in *Rickettsia* species may be explained by genome reduction. BMC Genomics. 2009;**10**(August):166

[19] Shpynov S, Pozdnichenko N, Gumenuk A. Approach for classification and taxonomy within family Rickettsiaceae based on the Formal Order Analysis. Microbes and Infection [Internet]. 2015;**17**(11-12):839-844. Available from: http://www.ncbi.nlm.nih.gov/pubmed/26423020

[20] Murray GGR, Weinert LA, Rhule EL, Welch JJ. The phylogeny of Rickettsia using different evolutionary signatures: How tree-like is bacterial evolution? Systems Biology [Internet]. 2016;**65**(2):265-279. Available from: http://www.ncbi.nlm.nih.gov/pubmed/26559010

[21] Andersson JO, Andersson SG. Genome degradation is an ongoing process in *Rickettsia*. Molecular Biology and Evolution. 1999;**16**(9):1178-1191

[22] Izzard L, Fuller A, Blacksell SD, Paris DH, Richards AL, Aukkanit N, et al. Isolation of a novel *Orientia* species (*O. chuto* sp. nov.) from a patient infected in Dubai. Journal of Clinical Microbiology. 2010;**48**(12):4404-4409

[23] Tamura A, Ohashi N, Urakami H, Miyamura S. Classification of *Rickettsia tsutsugamushi* in a new genus, *Orientia* gen. nov., as *Orientia tsutsugamushi* comb. nov. International Journal of Systematic Bacteriology. 1995;**45**(3):589-591

[24] Lee S-M, Kwon H-Y, Im J-H, Baek JH, Hwang S-S, Kang J-S, et al. *In vitro* activity of Tigecycline against *Orientia tsutsugamushi*. Yonsei Medical Journal. 2016;**57**(4):1034-1037

[25] Kelly DJ, Fuerst PA, Ching W-M, Richards AL. Scrub typhus: The geographic distribution of phenotypic and genotypic variants of *Orientia tsutsugamushi*. Clinical Infectious Diseases. 2009;**48**(Supplement 3):S203-S230

[26] Watt G, Parola P. Scrub typhus and tropical rickettsioses. Current Opinion in Infectious Diseases. 2003;**16**(5):429-436

[27] Zhang M, Zhao Z-T, Yang H-L, Zhang A-H, Xu X-Q, Meng X-P, et al. Molecular epidemiology of *Orientia tsutsugamushi* in chiggers and ticks from domestic rodents in Shandong, northern China. Parasites & Vectors. 2013;**6**(1):1-9

[28] Cosson JF, Galan M, Bard E, Razzauti M, Bernard M, Morand S, et al. Detection of *Orientia* sp. DNA in rodents from Asia, West Africa and Europe. Parasites & Vectors. 2015;**8**(1):1-4

[29] Blacksell SD, Luksameetanasan R, Kalambaheti T, Aukkanit N, Paris DH, McGready R, et al. Genetic typing of the 56-kDa type-specific antigen gene of contemporary *Orientia tsutsugamushi* isolates causing human scrub typhus at two sites in north-eastern and western Thailand. FEMS Immunology and Medical Microbiology. 2008;**52**(3):335-342

[30] Eisemann CS, Osterman JV. Identification of strain-specific and group-reactive antigenic determinants on the Karp, Gilliam and Kato strains of *Rickettsia tsutsugamushi*. The American Journal of Tropical Medicine and Hygiene. 1985;**34**(6):1173-1178

[31] Yang H-H, Huang I-T, Lin C-H, Chen T-Y, Chen L-K. New genotypes of *Orientia tsutsugamushi* isolated from humans in Eastern Taiwan. PLoS One. 2012;**7**(10):e46997

[32] Janardhanan J, Prakash JAJ, Abraham OC, Varghese GM. Comparison of a conventional and nested PCR for diagnostic confirmation and genotyping of *Orientia tsutsugamushi*. Diagnostic Microbiology and Infectious Disease. 2014;**79**(1):7-9

[33] Ruang-areerate T, Jeamwattanalert P, Rodkvamtook W, Richards AL, Sunyakumthorn P, Gaywee J. Genotype diversity and distribution of *Orientia tsutsugamushi* causing scrub typhus in Thailand. Journal of Clinical Microbiology. 2011;**49**(7):2584-2589

[34] Tamura A, Ohashi N, Koyama Y, Fukuhara M, Kawamori F, Otsuru M, et al. Characterization of *Orientia tsutsugamushi* isolated in Taiwan by immunofluorescence and restriction fragment length polymorphism analyses. FEMS Microbiology Letters. 1997; **150**(2):225-231

[35] Cho N-H, Kim H-R, Lee J-H, Kim S-Y, Kim J, Cha S, et al. The *Orientia tsutsugamushi* genome reveals massive proliferation of conjugative type IV secretion system and host-cell interaction genes. Proceedings of the National Academy of Sciences of the United States of America. 2007;**104**(19):7981-7986

[36] Nakayama K, Kurokawa K, Fukuhara M, Urakami H, Yamamoto S, Yamazaki K, et al. Genome comparison and phylogenetic analysis of *Orientia tsutsugamushi* strains. DNA Research: An International Journal for Rapid Publication of Reports on Genes and Genomes. 2010;**17**(5):281-291

[37] Nakayama K, Yamashita A, Kurokawa K, Morimoto T, Ogawa M, Fukuhara M, et al. The whole-genome sequencing of the obligate intracellular bacterium *Orientia tsutsugamushi* revealed massive gene amplification during reductive genome evolution. DNA Research. 2008;**15**(4):185-199

[38] Georgiades K, Merhej V, El Karkouri K, Raoult D, Pontarotti P. Gene gain and loss events in *Rickettsia* and *Orientia* species. Biology Direct. 2011;**6**:6

[39] Ogawa M, Shinkai-Ouchi F, Matsutani M, Uchiyama T, Hagiwara K, Hanada K, et al. Shotgun proteomics of *Orientia tsutsugamushi*. Clinical Microbiology and Infection [Internet]. 2009;**15**(Suppl. 2):239-240. Available from: http://dx.doi.org/10.1111/j.1469-0691.2008.02157.x

Chapter 6

Genomics of Apicomplexa

Fernando Martínez-Ocampo

Additional information is available at the end of the chapter

http://dx.doi.org/10.5772/intechopen.72633

Abstract

Apicomplexa is a eukaryotic phylum of intracellular parasites with more than 6000 species. Some of these single-celled parasites are important pathogens of livestock. At present, 128 genomes of phylum Apicomplexa have been reported in the GenBank database, of which 17 genomes belong to five genera that are pathogens of farm animals: *Babesia, Theileria, Eimeria, Neospora* and *Sarcocystis*. These 17 genomes are *Babesia bigemina* (five chromosomes), *Babesia divergens* (514 contigs) and *Babesia bovis* (four chromosomes and one apicoplast); *Theileria parva* (four chromosomes and one apicoplast), *Theileria annulata* (four chromosomes), *Theileria orientalis* (four chromosomes and one apicoplast) and *Theileria equi* (four chromosomes and one apicoplast); *Eimeria brunetti* (24,647 contigs), *Eimeria necatrix* (4667 contigs), *Eimeria tenella* (12,727 contigs), *Eimeria acervulina* (4947 contigs), *Eimeria maxima* (4570 contigs), *Eimeria mitis* (65,610 contigs) and *Eimeria praecox* (53,359 contigs); *Neospora caninum* (14 chromosomes); and *Sarcocystis neurona* strains SN1 (2862 contigs) and SN3 (3191 contigs). The study of these genomes allows us to understand their mechanisms of pathogenicity and identify genes that encode proteins as a possible vaccine antigen.

Keywords: Apicomplexa, genomics, parasitic protists, *Babesia, Theileria, Eimeria, Sarcocystis, Neospora*

1. Introduction

Apicomplexa (also called Apicomplexia) is a group of protists comprising a eukaryotic phylum of obligate intracellular parasites with more than 6000 described species [1]. Many of these cell single parasites are important pathogens of humans, domestic animals and livestock, with a health and economic relevance worldwide [2–5]. Apicomplexa microorganisms are intracellular eukaryotes thriving within another eukaryotic cell [6].

This phylum includes *Plasmodium falciparum* and four other *Plasmodium* species, the etiological agents for malaria in humans, a mosquito-transmitted and potentially deadly disease [6]. *Toxoplasma gondii* is a source of toxoplasmosis disease and congenital neurological birth defects (for example, encephalitis and ocular disease) in humans [7–9]. *Cryptosporidium* and *Cyclospora* parasites cause opportunistic human infections associated with immunosuppressive conditions (including AIDS) through contaminated food or water supplies [10, 11], while the invertebrate parasites of genus *Gregarina* are used as models for studying Apicomplexa motility [12].

Apicomplexa parasites infect a wide range of animals from mollusks to mammals [13]. Their life cycles involve only a single host, whereas others require sexual recombination in a vector species for transmission. The life cycle of these parasites has three stages: sporozoite (infective stage), merozoite (a result of asexual reproduction) and gametocyte (germ cells) [12]. These parasites are characterized by the presence of specific organelles (including rhoptries, micronemes and dense granules) involved in the establishment of an intracellular parasitophorous vacuole within the host cell [12].

A defined feature of these microorganisms is the presence of extracellular zoite forms that are usually motile and include an apical complex that gives the phylum its name [14]. With the exception of the genera *Cryptosporidium* and *Gregarina*, all species of the phylum Apicomplexa possess an apicoplast [12, 15–17].

The Apicomplexa parasites causing diseases of veterinary importance are *Babesia, Theileria, Eimeria, Neospora* and *Sarcocystis* [11, 18, 19]. This chapter focuses on genomics of these five genera.

2. Apicomplexa genome

2.1. Apicoplast genome

Twenty years ago, a remnant chloroplast, known as apicoplast, was discovered in *Plasmodium* [20–23]. This apicoplast lost the ability to perform photosynthesis, however, is an essential organelle, and its inhibition is lethal. The apicoplast arose from a secondary endosymbiosis event occurred where an ancestor to *Plasmodium* engulfed a photosynthetic alga [24–26]. This organelle is involved in critical metabolic pathways such as the biosynthesis of fatty acids and heme group degradation [27, 28]. Some of these metabolic pathways are considered as potential targets for antiparasitic drug designs [29, 30].

Like mitochondria, the apicoplast possesses its own genome [29, 31–37]. The apicoplast genome is ~35 kbp smaller than chloroplasts due to the absence of genes encoding proteins involved in photosynthesis. The genome of this plastid has been reduced and contains ribosomal (rRNA) and transfer RNA (tRNA) genes that play an important role in organelle replication [24]. The characteristics of the structure of apicoplast genomes have difficult comparisons with other plastids [20].

2.2. Apicomplexa genomes in GenBank

New drug targets identification, and novel antiparasitic therapeutics are necessary due to the emergence of parasite strains resistant to treatments available today [12, 38–40]. With the recent advancements in genome sequencing technologies, the research of new drug targets can be the focus on genomics analyses.

At present (August 2016), 123 complete and draft genomes of phylum Apicomplexa have been reported in the GenBank database (http://www.ncbi.nlm.nih.gov/genbank/), of which 17 genomes belong to five genera that are pathogens of farm animals: *Babesia, Theileria, Eimeria, Neospora,* and *Sarcocystis* (3, 4, 7, 1, and 2 genomes, respectively). The study and comparison of these genomes will allow us to understand pathogenicity mechanisms and identify genes and proteins with potential drug targets in order to develop novel antiparasitic compounds of veterinary importance.

3. Classification of phylum Apicomplexa

The National Center for Biotechnology Information (NCBI; http://www.ncbi.nlm.nih.gov/) divides the phylum Apicomplexa into two classes: Aconoidasida and Conoidasida (**Figure 1**). The class Aconoidasida is divided into two orders: Haemosporida and Piroplasmida

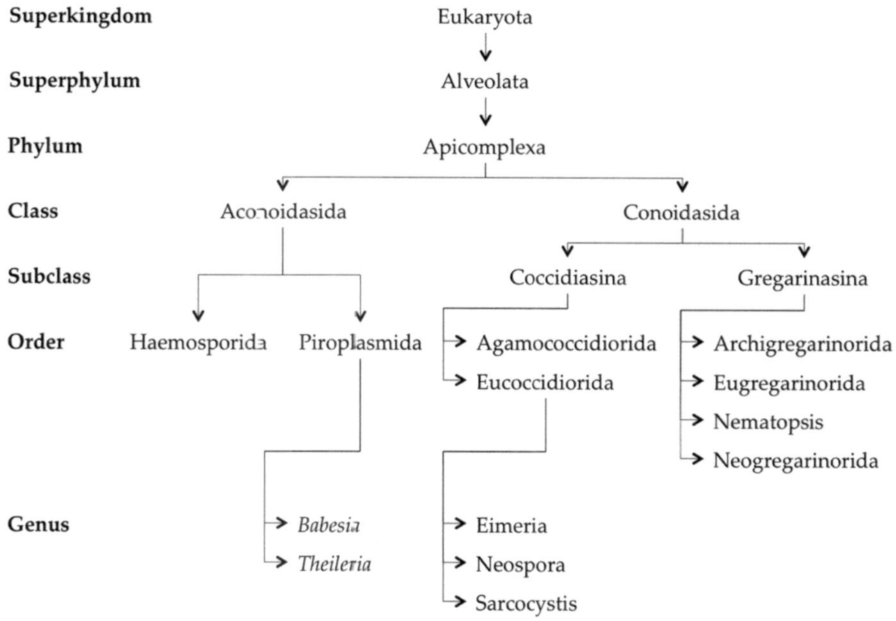

Figure 1. Classification of phylum Apicomplexa. Taxonomic categories are shown in bold (left). Only genera with veterinary importance are shown. The genera *Babesia* and *Theileria* belong to order Piroplasmida. The genera *Eimeria, Neospora* and *Sarcocystis* belong to order Eucoccidiorida.

(containing the genera *Babesia* and *Theileria*), while the class Conoidasida is divided into two subclasses: Coccidiasina (containing the genera *Eimeria, Neospora* and *Sarcocystis*, that belong to order Eucoccidiorida) and Gregarinasina (**Figure 1**).

It is estimated that subclass Coccidiasina separated from the class Aconoidasida ~705 million years ago [41, 42]. Moreover, in 2004, Douzery et al. calculated it as 495 million years ago [41–43].

4. *Babesia*

Babesia is a genus of intracellular protozoa that cause babesiosis. These parasites are transmitted by ticks and infect erythrocytes in their mammalian hosts. Babesiosis was first described in sheep and cattle in 1888 by Victor Babes, in honor of which is called the genus [44] and is characterized by hemolytic anemia and fever, with occasional hemoglobinuria and death [45].

The genus *Babesia* includes over 100 species that are highly specific for their hosts. Only a few *Babesia* species cause infections in humans, especially immunocompromised individuals. Most cases identified in humans are caused by *Babesia microti* and *Babesia divergens*, parasites of rodents and cattle, respectively [44, 46, 47].

Species affecting animals are: *Babesia bigemina, Babesia major, Babesia divergens* and *Babesia bovis* that infect cattle [44, 48–51]; *Babesia ovis* and *Babesia motasi* cause infections in sheep [44, 52, 53]; and *Babesia equi* and *Babesia caballi* cause infections in horses [44, 54].

Three genomes of *Babesia* species have been reported in the GenBank database. The *B. bigemina* strain Bond genome is 13,840,936 bp of total length divided into five chromosomes (2.5, 2.8, 3.5, 0.9 and 0.5 Mbp; GenBank accession number from NC_027216.1 to NC_027220.1, respectively). The *B. divergens* strain Rouen 1987 genome is 10,797,556 bp divided into 514 contigs (GenBank accession number CCSG00000000.1).

B. bovis strain T2Bo genome is 8,179,706 bp divided into four chromosomes (1.2, 1.7, 2.6 and 2.6 Mbp, respectively) and one apicoplast (35,107 bp, GenBank accession number NC_011395.1). The chromosomes I and IV of *B. bovis* genome are divided into seven and three contigs, respectively; chromosomes II and III GenBank accession numbers are NC_010574.1 and NC_010575.1, respectively.

4.1. *Babesia bovis* genome

In 2007, Brayton et al. reported the analysis of comparative genomic between *B. bovis, Theileria parva* and *P. falciparum* genomes [33]. The *B. bovis* genome has 3671 protein-coding genes and 41.8% of GC content, an analysis of enzymatic pathways revealed a reduced metabolic potential. The results of comparative genomic showed that *B. bovis* genome (8.2 Mbp) is similar in size to that of *T. parva* (8.3 Mbp) [34] and *Theileria annulata* (8.35 Mbp) [55], the smallest Apicomplexa genomes sequenced to date.

In contrast, *B. bovis* and *P. falciparum*, which have similar clinical and pathological features, have major differences in genome size (8.2 and 22.8 Mbp, respectively) and chromosome number (4 and 14, respectively). Additionally, many stage-specific and immunologically important genes from *P. falciparum* are absent in *B. bovis* [33]. The *B. bovis* genome sequence has allowed analyses of the polymorphic variant erythrocyte surface antigen protein (*ves1* gene and discovery of the novel *smorf* gene family) that are postulated to play a role in cytoadhesion and immune evasion (similar to *var.* genes of *P. falciparum*). The ~150 *ves1* genes are distributed in clusters throughout each chromosome [33]. Finally, comparative analyses have identified several novel vaccine candidates into B. bovis genome, including homologs of p36 and Pf12 (*P. falciparum*); p67 and four of six proteins (*T. parva*) targeted by $CD8^+$ cytotoxic T cells [33].

Brayton et al. also reported that the *B. bovis* apicoplast genome is 33 kbp of total length and encodes 32 putative protein coding genes, 25 tRNA genes, and small and large subunit rRNA genes. This organelle genome displays similarities in size and gene content to apicoplasts of *Eimeria tenella, P. falciparum, T. parva* and *T. gondii* [33, 35, 56]. The *B. bovis* apicoplast genome has 78.2% of AT content (21.8% of GC content) [33].

5. *Theileria*

The genus *Theileria* infects leukocytes [57], and they are the only eukaryotic pathogens known to transform lymphocytes [11]. These parasites infect a wide range of both domestic and wild animals and are transmitted by Ixodid ticks of the genera *Amblyomma, Haemaphysalis, Hyalomma* and *Rhipicephalus* [58, 59]. *Theileria* parasites can be grouped into schizont transforming (*T. parva, T. annulata* and *Theileria lestoquardi*) [60–62] and nontransforming (*Theileria orientalis*) species [63, 64]. The uncontrolled proliferation of schizonts results in the pathologies associated with corridor disease and East Coast fever (*T. parva*), tropical theileriosis (*T. annulata*) in cattle and malignant theileriosis (*T. lestoquardi*) in goats and sheep [59, 65].

T. orientalis (frequently been referred to as *T. sergenti* [66]) causes bovine piroplasmosis [67–69] and can generate anemia and icterus in cattle but rarely cause fatal disease [64]. *T. orientalis* is classified into two major genotypes: the Chitose (throughout the world) and Ikeda (eastern Asian countries) types [70]. Finally, equine piroplasmosis of horses, mules, donkeys, and zebras is caused by *Theileria equi* [71]. *T. equi* has been renamed several times [72], and molecular phylogenetic analyses indicate an intermediate position between *B. bovis* and *Theileria* spp. [73, 74].

Four genomes of *Theileria* species have been reported in the GenBank database. The *T. parva* strain Muguga genome is 8,347,606 bp divided into four chromosomes (2.5, 2.0, 1.9 and 1.9 Mbp) and one apicoplast (39,579 bp, GenBank accession number NC_007758.1). The chromosomes I and II of *T. parva* genome have the GenBank accession number NC_007344.1 and NC_007345.1, respectively, while the chromosomes III and IV are divided into four and two contigs, respectively. The *T. annulata* strain Ankara isolate clone C9 genome is 8,358,425 bp divided into four chromosomes (2.6, 2.0, 1.9 and 1.8 Mbp; GenBank accession number

NC_011129.1, NC_011099.1, NC_011100.1 and NC_011098.1, respectively). The *T. orientalis* strain Shintoku (Ikeda type) genome is 9,010,364 bp divided into four chromosomes (2.7, 2.2, 2.0 and 2.0 Mbp; GenBank accession number from NC_025260.1 to NC_025263.1, respectively) and one apicoplast (24,173 bp into one contig).

Finally, the *T. equi* strain WA genome is 11,674,479 bp divided into four chromosomes (3.7, 2.3, 2.1 and 3.5 Mbp) and one apicoplast (47,880 bp into one contig). The chromosomes I and III of *T. equi* genome have the GenBank accession number NC_021366.1 and NC_021367.1, respectively, while the chromosomes II and IV are divided into two and six contigs, respectively.

5.1. *Theileria parva* genome

The complete genome sequence of *T. parva* was reported in 2005 [34]. *T. parva* genome has 4035 protein encoding genes (20% fewer than *P. falciparum*) and 34.1% of GC content. Putative functions were assigned to 38% of the predicted proteins. Like *P. falciparum*, the four chromosomes of *T. parva* contain one extremely A + T-rich region (>97%) about 3 kbp in length that may be the centromere [34]. Unlike *P. falciparum*, *T. parva* genome contains two identical, unlinked 5.8S-18S-28S rRNA units, which suggest that it does not possess functionally distinct ribosomes [75]. The infection of T and B lymphocytes by *T. parvum* results in a reversible transformed phenotype with uncontrolled proliferation of host cells that remain persistently infected. Parasite proteins that may modulate host cell phenotype are described by [55]. Telomeres of *T. parvum* have a conserved (~140 bp) sequence adjacent to the telomeric repeat and several subtelomeric regions exhibit 70–100% sequence similarity [34, 76]. The apicoplast genome of *T. parva* differs from *P. falciparum* in that all of its genes are transcribed in the same direction, and 26 of the 44 protein-coding genes share 27–61% sequence similarity with proteins encoded by the *P. falciparum* apicoplast genome [34].

5.2. *Theileria annulata* genome

The *T. annulata* genome sequence was also reported in 2005 [55]. The nuclear genome of *T. annulata* is similar in size (8.35 Mbp) to that of *T. parva* (8.3 Mbp). *T. annulata* genome has 3792 protein encoding genes (243 genes fewer than *T. parva*), 49 tRNA and 5 rRNA genes, and 32.54% of GC content. In addition, 3265 orthologous genes were predicted between *T. annulata* and *T. parva* genomes. Pain et al. predicted 3265 orthologous genes between the *T. annulata* and *T. parva* genomes. Additionally, 34 (*T. annulata*) and 60 (*T. parva*) genes are single-copy genes and their functions have been not described [55].

The parasite genes involved in host-cell transformation require a signal peptide or a specific host-targeting signal sequence. Some candidates include TashAT and SuAT protein families in *T. annulata* [77, 78] and related host nuclear proteins (TpHNs protein family) in *T. parva*. A cluster of 17 SuAT1 and TashAT-like genes was identified in the *T. annulata* genome [55].

5.3. *Theileria orientalis* genome

In 2012, Hayashida et al. reported the comparative genomic analyses between *T. orientalis*, *T. parva*, *T. annulata* and *B. bovis*. The genome size of *T. orientalis* (9 Mbp) is approximately

8% larger than the reported genome sizes of *T. parva* (8.3 Mbp), *T. annulata* (8.35 Mbp) and *B. bovis* (8.2 Mbp). The number of predicted protein-coding (3995) genes identified in *T. orientalis* is similar to that found in *T. parva* (4035). The GC content of the *T. orientalis* genome (41.6%) is higher than *T. parva* and *T. annulata* (34.1 and 32.5%, respectively) but similar to *B. bovis* (41.8%). Unlike *T. parva* and *T. annulata, T. orientalis* does not induce uncontrolled proliferation of infected leukocytes and multiplies predominantly within infected erythrocytes [79]. *T. orientalis* is the first genome sequence of a nontransforming *Theileria* species that occupies a phylogenetic position close to that of the transforming species [79].

5.4. *Theileria equi* genome

The *T. equi* genome sequence was reported in 2012 [80]. *T. equi* genome size (11.6 Mbp) is larger than *T. parva* (8.3 Mbp), *T. annulata* (8.35 Mbp), *T. orientalis* (9 Mbp) and *B. bovis* (8.2 Mbp). *T. equi* genome has two rRNA operons, 46 tRNA genes and 5330 nuclear protein coding genes, ~25% greater than found for *T. parva, T. annulata* and *B. bovis*. Furthermore, *T. equi* genome contains 1985 unique genes, and 366 and 137 homologs of genes found only in the two *Theileria* spp. or *B. bovis*, respectively. The apicoplast genome of *T. Equi* has 43 unidirectionally coding sequences, which includes each of the 20 tRNA, and two rRNA genes are present [80].

6. *Eimeria*

Eimeria is a genus that includes species capable of causing the disease coccidiosis in cattle and poultry. *Eimeria* parasites exhibit immense diversity in host range including mammals, birds, reptiles, fish and amphibians [81–86]. It is estimated that there are many thousands of *Eimeria* species [87]. Coccidiosis is primarily associated with enteric disease with few exceptions [88–90]. The avian coccidiosis can be subdivided into hemorrhagic and malabsorptive pathologies related to *Eimeria brunetti*, *Eimeria necatrix* and *Eimeria tenella*; or *Eimeria acervulina, Eimeria maxima, Eimeria mitis* and *Eimeria praecox*, respectively [91]. *E. tenella* is among the most pathogenic avian parasites causing weight loss, reduced feed efficiency, reduced egg production and death [92]. The total loss is estimated at around USD 2.4 billion annually [93], including the costs of control and prevention worldwide.

Seven genomes of *Eimeria* species have been reported in the GenBank database. The *E. brunetti* strain Houghton genome is 66,890,165 bp divided into 24,647 contigs (GenBank accession number CBUX000000000.1). The *E. necatrix* strain Houghton genome is 55,007,932 bp divided into 4667 contigs (GenBank accession number CBUZ000000000.1). The *E. tenella* strain Houghton genome is 51,859,607 bp divided into 12,727 contigs (GenBank accession number CBUW000000000.1). The *E. acervulina* strain Houghton genome is 45,830,609 bp divided into 4947 contigs (GenBank accession number CBUS000000000.1). The *E. maxima* strain Weybridge genome is 45,975,062 bp divided into 4570 contigs (GenBank accession number CBUY000000000.1). The *E. mitis* strain Houghton genome is 60,415,144 bp divided into 65,610 contigs (GenBank accession number CBUT000000000.1). *E. praecox* strain Houghton genome is 60,083,328 bp divided into 53,359 contigs (CBUU000000000.1).

E. tenella strain Houghton was isolated in the United Kingdom in 1949. The *E. tenella* genome size is ~60 Mbp with a GC content of ~53%. Its molecular karyotype comprises 14 chromosomes of between 1 and >6 Mbp, and the genome is available in http://www.sanger.ac.uk/Projects/E_tenella/. Moreover, parallel projects have been undertaken to generate the complete sequences of chromosomes I (~1 Mbp) and II (~1.2 Mbp), which are associated with resistance to the anticoccidial drug arprinocid and precocious development, respectively [94]. In 2007, Ling et al. reported the sequencing and analysis of the first chromosome of *E. tenella* [95]. The chromosome I of *E. tenella* is 1,347,714 pb of total length and has the GenBank accession number AM269894.1.

7. *Neospora*

The genus *Neospora* is constituted by only two species: *Neospora caninum* and *Neospora hughesi*. *N. caninum* is the etiologic agent of the disease neosporosis and is a close relative of *T. gondii* [96]. They share many common morphological and biological features [97]. *Neospora* parasite appears not to be zoonotic, having a more restricted host range [98, 99], and shows a striking capacity for highly efficient vertical transmission in bovines [100]. *N. caninum* is one of the leading causes of infectious bovine abortion [101, 102].

Only one genome of *N. caninum* strain Liverpool has been reported in the GenBank database. This genome has 57,547,420 bp of total length divided into 14 chromosomes: Ia (2,288,409 bp), Ib (1,908,326 bp), II (2,170,133 bp), III (2,139,717 bp), IV (2,317,323 bp), V (2,735,753 bp), VI (3,360,651 bp), VIIa (3,947,736 bp), VIIb (4,923,984 bp), VIII (6,723,156 bp), IX (5,490,906 bp), X (6,985,512 bp), XI (6,081,843 bp) and XII (6,473,971 bp); GenBank accession number from NC_018385.1 to NC_018398.1.

8. *Sarcocystis*

More than 150 species of *Sarcocystis* have an indirect life cycle. They require both an intermediate and a final host, usually a herbivorous and a carnivorous vertebrate animal, respectively [103]. For this transition, *Sarcocystis* species produce infectious tissue cysts surrounded by glycosylated cyst walls that are largely restricted to muscle. Ingestion of tissue cysts through predation by the final hosts propagates the life cycle [104]. All vertebrates, including mammals, some birds, reptiles and possibly fish, are intermediate hosts to at least one *Sarcocystis* species [105, 106]. Final hosts include carnivores or omnivores, such as humans, some reptiles and raptorial birds [107].

Sarcocystis species are the causal agents of Sarcocystosis, a disease typically asymptomatic but can be associated with myositis, diarrhea or infection of the central nervous system [104]. Some species of *Sarcocystis* that infect farm animals (such as cattle, sheep and horses) cause fever, lethargy, poor growth, reduced milk production, abortion and death [107].

Sarcocysti cruzi, *Sarcocysti hirsuta* and *Sarcocysti hominis* used cattle as intermediate hosts, and canids, felids and humans as final hosts, respectively [108]. Additionally, *Sarcocysti sinensis* also used cattle as intermediate host [109], but its final host remains to be elucidated [110]. *S. hominis* causes gastrointestinal malaise [108] and *S. sinensis* may also elicit symptoms in humans [111].

Sarcocysti neurona is the causal agent of equine protozoal myeloencephalitis [106]. This disease destroys neural tissue and can be fatal to horses, marine mammals and several other mammals. *S. neurona* also infects many mammals asymptomatically [104]. Furthermore, three *Sarcocystis* species have been identified from pigs: *Sarcocysti miescheriana*, *Sarcocysti porcifelis* and *Sarcocysti suihominis* [112]. In 2015, Blazejewski et al. reported the first genome sequence of *S. neurona* strain SN1 [104].

Two genomes of *S. neurona* strains have been reported in the GenBank database. The *S. neurona* strain SN3 clone E1 genome is 124,404,968 bp divided into 3191 contigs (GenBank accession number JAQE00000000.1). *S. neurona* strain SN1 genome is 130,023,008 bp divided into 2862 contigs (GenBank accession number JXWP00000000.1). *S. neurona* strain SN1 was isolated from an otter that died of protozoal encephalitis [113]. The apicoplast genome architectures of *S. neurona* strains SN1 and SN3 are highly similar to those of *Toxoplasma gondii* and *Plasmodium falciparum* [104]. *S. neurona* strains SN1 and SN3 are the first genomes reported in the genus *Sarcocystis*. These genomes are more than twice the size of other sequenced coccidian genomes.

Acknowledgements

This work was supported by CONACyT scholarship 293,552.

Author details

Fernando Martínez-Ocampo

Address all correspondence to: fernando.martinezo@uaem.mx

Laboratory of Ecogenomic Studies, Biotechnology Research Center (CEIB), Autonomous University of the State of Morelos (UAEM), Cuernavaca, Morelos, Mexico

References

[1] Adl SM, Leander BS, Simpson AGB, Archibald JM, Anderson OR, Bass D, et al. Diversity, nomenclature, and taxonomy of protists. Systematic Biology(England). 2007 Aug;**56**(4): 684-689

[2] Battle KE, Gething PW, Elyazar IRF, Moyes CL, Sinka ME, Howes RE, et al. The global public health significance of Plasmodium vivax. Advances in Parasitology(England). 2012;**80**:1-111

[3] Checkley W, White ACJ, Jaganath D, Arrowood MJ, Chalmers RM, Chen X-M, et al. A review of the global burden, novel diagnostics, therapeutics, and vaccine targets for cryptosporidium. The Lancet Infectious Diseases (United States). 2015 Jan;**15**(1):85-94

[4] Morrison WI. The aetiology, pathogenesis and control of theileriosis in domestic animals. Revue Scientifique Et Technique (France). 2015 Aug;**34**(2):599-611

[5] Torgerson PR, Mastroiacovo P. The global burden of congenital toxoplasmosis: A systematic review. Bulletin of the World Health Organization (Switzerland). 2013 Jul;**91**(7):501-508

[6] Seeber F, Steinfelder S. Recent advances in understanding apicomplexan parasites. F1000Research (England). 2016;**5**

[7] Belanger F, Derouin F, Grangeot-Keros L, Meyer L. Incidence and risk factors of toxoplasmosis in a cohort of human immunodeficiency virus-infected patients: 1988-1995. HEMOCO and SEROCO Study Groups. Clinical Infectious Diseases (United States). 1999 Mar;**28**(3):575-581

[8] Schluter D, Daubener W, Schares G, Gross U, Pleyer U, Luder C. Animals are key to human toxoplasmosis. International Journal of Medical Microbiology (Germany). 2014 Oct;**304**(7):917-929

[9] Havelaar AH, Kirk MD, Torgerson PR, Gibb HJ, Hald T, Lake RJ, et al. World health organization global estimates and regional comparisons of the burden of foodborne disease in 2010. PLoS Med (United States). 2015 Dec;**12**(12):e1001923

[10] Hunter PR, Nichols G. Epidemiology and clinical features of Cryptosporidium infection in immunocompromised patients. Clinical Microbiology Reviews (United States). 2002 Jan;**15**(1):145-154

[11] Roos DS. Genetics. Themes and variations in apicomplexan parasite biology. Science. (United States). 2005 Jul;**309**(5731):72-73

[12] Wasmuth J, Daub J, Peregrin-Alvarez JM, Finney CAM, Parkinson J. The origins of apicomplexan sequence innovation. Genome Research (United States). 2009 Jul;**19**(7):1202-1213

[13] Cavalier-Smith T. Kingdom protozoa and its 18 phyla. Microbiological Reviews (United States). 1993 Dec;**57**(4):953-994

[14] Sibley LD. Intracellular parasite invasion strategies. Science (United States). 2004 Apr; **304**(5668):248-253

[15] Zhu G, Marchewka MJ, Keithly JS. Cryptosporidium parvum appears to lack a plastid genome. Microbiology (England). 2000 Feb;**146**(Pt 2:315-321)

[16] Fast NM, Kissinger JC, Roos DS, Keeling PJ. Nuclear-encoded, plastid-targeted genes suggest a single common origin for apicomplexan and dinoflagellate plastids. Molecular Biology and Evolution (United States). 2001 Mar;**18**(3):418-426

[17] Toso MA, Omoto CK. Gregarina niphandrodes may lack both a plastid genome and organelle. The Journal of Eukaryotic Microbiology (United States). 2007;**54**(1):66-72

[18] Graat EA, Ploeger HW, Henken AM, De Vries Reilingh G, Noordhuizen JP, Van Beek PN. Effects of initial litter contamination level with Eimeria acervulina on population dynamics and production characteristics in broilers. Veterinary Parasitology (Netherlands). 1996 Oct;**65**(3-4):223-232

[19] Dubey JP. Recent advances in Neospora and neosporosis. Veterinary Parasitology (Netherlands). 1999 Aug;**84**(3-4):349-367

[20] Wilson RJ, Denny PW, Preiser PR, Rangachari K, Roberts K, Roy A, et al. Complete gene map of the plastid-like DNA of the malaria parasite Plasmodium falciparum. Journal of Molecular Biology(England). 1996 Aug;**261**(2):155-172

[21] Gardner MJ, Williamson DH, Wilson RJ. A circular DNA in malaria parasites encodes an RNA polymerase like that of prokaryotes and chloroplasts. Molecular and Biochemical Parasitology (Netherlands). 1991 Jan;**44**(1):115-123

[22] Howe CJ. Plastid origin of an extrachromosomal DNA molecule from Plasmodium, the causative agent of malaria. Journal of Theoretical Biology (England). 1992 Sep; **158**(2):199-205

[23] McFadden GI, Reith ME, Munholland J, Lang-Unnasch N. Plastid in human parasites. Nature (England). 1996;**381**:482

[24] Nisbet RER, McKenzie JL. Transcription of the apicoplast genome. Molecular and Biochemical Parasitology. 2016 Jul

[25] Kohler S, Delwiche CF, Denny PW, Tilney LG, Webster P, Wilson RJ, et al. A plastid of probable green algal origin in Apicomplexan parasites. Science (United States). 1997 Mar;**275**(5305):1485-1489

[26] Janouskovec J, Horak A, Obornik M, Lukes J, Keeling PJ. A common red algal origin of the apicomplexan, dinoflagellate, and heterokont plastids. Proceedings of the National Academy of Sciences of the United States of America (United States). 2010 Jun;**107**(24):10949-10954

[27] Ralph SA, van Dooren GG, Waller RF, Crawford MJ, Fraunholz MJ, Foth BJ, et al. Tropical infectious diseases: Metabolic maps and functions of the Plasmodium falciparum apicoplast. Nature Reviews. Microbiology 2004 Mar;**2**(3):203-216

[28] Waller RF, McFadden GI. The apicoplast: A review of the derived plastid of apicomplexan parasites. Current Issues in Molecular Biology (England). 2005 Jan;**7**(1):57-79

[29] Huang Y, He L, Hu J, He P, He J, Yu L, et al. Characterization and annotation of Babesia orientalis apicoplast genome. Parasites and Vectors (England). 2015;**8**:543

[30] Aboulaila M, Munkhjargal T, Sivakumar T, Ueno A, Nakano Y, Yokoyama M, et al. Apicoplast-targeting antibacterials inhibit the growth of Babesia parasites. Antimicrobial Agents and Chemotherapy (United States). 2012 Jun;**56**(6):3196-3206

[31] Imura T, Sato S, Sato Y, Sakamoto D, Isobe T, Murata K, et al. The apicoplast genome of Leucocytozoon caulleryi, a pathogenic apicomplexan parasite of the chicken. Parasitology Research (Germany). 2014 Mar;**113**(3):823-828

[32] Lau AOT, McElwain TF, Brayton KA, Knowles DP, Roalson EH. Babesia bovis: a comprehensive phylogenetic analysis of plastid-encoded genes supports green algal origin of apicoplasts. Experimental Parasitology (United States). 2009 Nov;**123**(3):236-243

[33] Brayton KA, Lau AOT, Herndon DR, Hannick L, Kappmeyer LS, Berens SJ, et al. Genome sequence of Babesia bovis and comparative analysis of apicomplexan hemoprotozoa. PLoS Pathogens (United States). 2007 Oct;**3**(10):1401-1413

[34] Gardner MJ, Bishop R, Shah T, de Villiers EP, Carlton JM, Hall N, et al. Genome sequence of Theileria parva, a bovine pathogen that transforms lymphocytes. Science (United States). 2005 Jul;**309**(5731):134-137

[35] Cai X, Fuller AL, McDougald LR, Zhu G. Apicoplast genome of the coccidian Eimeria tenella. Gene (Netherlands). 2003 Dec;**321**:39-46

[36] Williamson DH, Denny PW, Moore PW, Sato S, McCready S, Wilson RJ. The in vivo conformation of the plastid DNA of Toxoplasma gondii: implications for replication. Journal of Molecular Biology. 2001 Feb;**306**(2):159-168

[37] Tang K, Guo Y, Zhang L, Rowe LA, Roellig DM, Frace MA, et al. Genetic similarities between Cyclospora cayetanensis and cecum-infecting avian Eimeria spp. in apicoplast and mitochondrial genomes. Parasites & Vectors (England). 2015;**8**:358

[38] Aspinall T V, Joynson DHM, Guy E, Hyde JE, Sims PFG. The molecular basis of sulfonamide resistance in Toxoplasma gondii and implications for the clinical management of toxoplasmosis. The Journal of Infectious Diseases (United States). 2002 Jun;**185**(11):1637-1643

[39] Trouiller P, Olliaro P, Torreele E, Orbinski J, Laing R, Ford N. Drug development for neglected diseases: a deficient market and a public-health policy failure. Lancet (London, England). 2002 Jun;**359**(9324):2188-2194

[40] White NJ. Antimalarial drug resistance. The Journal of Clinical Investigation. 2004;**113**:1084-1092

[41] Shanmugasundram A, Gonzalez-Galarza FF, Wastling JM, Vasieva O, Jones AR. Library of Apicomplexan Metabolic Pathways: a manually curated database for metabolic pathways of apicomplexan parasites. Nucleic Acids Research (England). 2013 Jan;**41**(Database issue):D706-D713

[42] Hedges SB, Dudley J, Kumar S. TimeTree: A public knowledge-base of divergence times among organisms. Bioinformatics (England). 2006 Dec;**22**(23):2971-2972

[43] Douzery EJP, Snell EA, Bapteste E, Delsuc F, Philippe H. The timing of eukaryotic evolution: Does a relaxed molecular clock reconcile proteins and fossils? Proceedings of the National Academy of Sciences of the United States of America (United States). 2004 Oct;**101**(43):15386-15391

[44] Beugnet F, Moreau Y. Babesiosis. Revue Scientifique Et Technique (France). 2015 Aug; **34**(2):627-639

[45] Mosqueda J, Olvera-Ramirez A, Aguilar-Tipacamu G, Canto GJ. Current advances in detection and treatment of babesiosis. Current Medicinal Chemistry (Netherlands). 2012;**19**(10):1504-1518

[46] Hunfeld K-P, Hildebrandt A, Gray JS. Babesiosis: Recent insights into an ancient disease. International Journal for Parasitology (England). 2008 Sep;**38**(11):1219-1237

[47] Cassini R, Bonoli C, Montarsi F, Tessarin C, Marcer F, Galuppi R. Detection of Babesia EU1 in Ixodes ricinus ticks in northern Italy. Veterinary Parasitology (Netherlands). 2010 Jul;**171**(1-2):151-154

[48] Doyle RL, Da Silva AS, Oliveira CB, Franca RT, Carvalho FB, Abdalla FH, et al. Cholinesterases as markers of the inflammatory process associated oxidative stress in cattle infected by Babesia bigemina. Comparative Immunology, Microbiology & Infectious Diseases (England). 2016 Jun;**46**:1-6

[49] Purnell RE, Brocklesby DW, Stark AJ. Protection of cattle against Babesia major by the inoculation of irradiated piroplasms. Research in Veterinary Science (England). 1978 Nov;**25**(3):388-390

[50] Cuesta I, Gonzalez LM, Estrada K, Grande R, Zaballos A, Lobo CA, et al. High-Quality Draft Genome Sequence of Babesia divergens, the Etiological Agent of Cattle and Human Babesiosis. Genome Announcements (United States). 2014;**2**(6)

[51] Yang C, Liu J, Li A, Li Y, Liu A, Xie J, et al. Evaluating the Babesia bovis infection of cattle in China with enzyme-linked immunosorbent assay (ELISA). Acta Parasitologica (Poland). 2015 Dec;**60**(4):721-726

[52] Erster O, Roth A, Wollkomirsky R, Leibovich B, Savitzky I, Zamir S, et al. Quantitative analysis of Babesia ovis infection in sheep and ticks. Veterinary Parasitology (Netherlands). 2016 May **221**:39-45

[53] Alani AJ, Herbert I V. The pathogenesis of Babesia motasi (Wales) infection in sheep. Veterinary Parasitology (Netherlands). 1988 Mar;**27**(3-4):209-220

[54] Xu Y, Zhang S, Huang X, Bayin C, Xuan X, Igarashi I, et al. Seroepidemiologic studies on Babesia equi and Babesia caballi infections in horses in Jilin province of China. The Journal of Veterinary Medical Science (Japan). 2003 Sep;**65**(9):1015-1017

[55] Pain A, Renauld H, Berriman M, Murphy L, Yeats CA, Weir W, et al. Genome of the host-cell transforming parasite Theileria annulata compared with T. parva. Science (United States). 2005 Jul;**309**(5731):131-133

[56] Williamson DH, Gardner MJ, Preiser P, Moore DJ, Rangachari K, Wilson RJ. The evolutionary origin of the 35 kb circular DNA of Plasmodium falciparum: new evidence supports a possible rhodophyte ancestry. Molecular Genetics and Genomics (Germany). 1994 Apr;**243**(2):249-252

[57] Uilenberg G. Babesia. A historical overview. Veterinary Parasitology (Netherlands). 2006 May;**138**(1-2):3-10

[58] Mans BJ, Pienaar R, Latif AA. A review of Theileria diagnostics and epidemiology. International Journal for Parasitology: Parasites and Wildlife (England). 2015 Apr; **4**(1):104-118

[59] Bishop R, Musoke A, Morzaria S, Gardner M, Nene V. Theileria: Intracellular protozoan parasites of wild and domestic ruminants transmitted by ixodid ticks. Parasitology (England). 2004;**129** Suppl:S271–S283

[60] Irvin AD, Brown CG, Kanhai GK, Stagg DA. Comparative growth of bovine lymphosarcoma cells and lymphoid cells infected with Theileria parva in athymic (nude) mice. Nature (England). 1975 Jun;**255**(5511):713-714

[61] Brown CG. Control of tropical theileriosis (Theileria annulata infection) of cattle. Parassitologia (Italy). 1990 Apr;**32**(1):23-31

[62] Hooshmand-Rad P, Hawa NJ. Malignant theileriosis of sheep and goats. Tropical Animal Health and Production. 1973;**5**(2):97-102

[63] Sivakumar T, Hayashida K, Sugimoto C, Yokoyama N. Evolution and genetic diversity of Theileria. Infection, Genetics and Evolution (Netherlands). 2014 Oct;**27**:250-263

[64] Onuma M, Kakuda T, Sugimoto C. Theileria parasite infection in East Asia and control of the disease. Comparative Immunology, Microbiology and Infectious Diseases (England). 1998 Jul;**21**(3):165-177

[65] McKeever DJ. Bovine immunity—A driver for diversity in Theileria parasites? Trends in Parasitology. 2009 Jun;**25**(6):269-276

[66] Uilenberg G. Theileria sergenti. Vol. 175. Netherlands: Veterinary parasitology; 2011 p. 386

[67] Shimizu S, Yoshiura N, Mizomoto T, Kondou Y. Theileria sergenti infection in dairy cattle. The Journal of Veterinary Medical Science (Japan). 1992 Apr;**54**(2):375-377

[68] Uilenberg G, Perie NM, Spanjer AA, Franssen FF. Theileria orientalis, a cosmopolitan blood parasite of cattle: Demonstration of the schizont stage. Research in Veterinary Science. 1985 May;**38**(3):352-360

[69] Fujisaki K, Kawazu S, Kamio T. The taxonomy of the bovine Theileria spp. Parasitology Today (England). 1994 Jan;**10**(1):31-33

[70] Kubota S, Sugimoto C, Onuma M. Population dynamics of Theileria sergenti in persistently infected cattle and vector ticks analysed by a polymerase chain reaction. Parasitology (England). 1996 May;**112** (Pt 5:437-442)

[71] Ueti MW, Palmer GH, Scoles GA, Kappmeyer LS, Knowles DP. Persistently Infected horses are reservoirs for intrastadial tick-borne transmission of the Apicomplexan parasite Babesia equi. Infection and Immunity. 2008;**76**:3525-3529

[72] Mehlhorn H, Schein E. Redescription of Babesia equi Laveran, 1901 as Theileria equi Mehlhorn, Schein 1998. Parasitology Research (Germany). 1998 Jun;**84**(6):467-475

[73] Allsopp MT, Cavalier-Smith T, De Waal DT, Allsopp BA. Phylogeny and evolution of the piroplasms. Parasitology (England). 1994 Feb;**108** (Pt 2:147-152)

[74] Allsopp MTEP, Allsopp BA. Molecular sequence evidence for the reclassification of some Babesia species. Annals of the New York Academy of Sciences (United States). 2006 Oct;**1081**:509-517

[75] Gunderson JH, Sogin ML, Wollett G, Hollingdale M, de la Cruz VF, Waters AP, et al. Structurally distinct, stage-specific ribosomes occur in Plasmodium. Science (United States). 1987 Nov;**238**(4829):933-937

[76] Sohanpal B, Wasawo D, Bishop R. Cloning of telomere-associated DNA using single-specific-primer polymerase chain reaction provides evidence for a conserved sequence directly adjacent to Theileria parva telomeric repeats. Gene (Netherlands). 2000 Sep;**255**(2):401-409

[77] Shiels BR, McKellar S, Katzer F, Lyons K, Kinnaird J, Ward C, et al. A Theileria annulata DNA binding protein localized to the host cell nucleus alters the phenotype of a bovine macrophage cell line. Eukaryotic Cell (United States). 2004 Apr;**3**(2):495-505

[78] Swan DG, Phillips K, Tait A, Shiels BR. Evidence for localisation of a Theileria parasite AT hook DNA-binding protein to the nucleus of immortalised bovine host cells. Molecular and Biochemical Parasitology (Netherlands). 1999 Jun;**101**(1-2):117-129

[79] Hayashida K, Hara Y, Abe T, Yamasaki C, Toyoda A, Kosuge T, et al. Comparative genome analysis of three eukaryotic parasites with differing abilities to transform leukocytes reveals key mediators of Theileria-induced leukocyte transformation. MBio (United States). 2012;**3**(5):e00204-e00212

[80] Kappmeyer LS, Thiagarajan M, Herndon DR, Ramsay JD, Caler E, Djikeng A, et al. Comparative genomic analysis and phylogenetic position of Theileria equi. BMC Genomics (England). 2012;**13**:603

[81] Jirku M, Jirku M, Obornik M, Lukes J, Modry D. A model for taxonomic work on homoxenous coccidia: redescription, host specificity, and molecular phylogeny of Eimeria ranae Dobell, 1909, with a review of anuran-host Eimeria (Apicomplexa: Eimeriorina). The Journal of Eukaryotic Microbiology (United States). 2009;**56**(1):39-51

[82] Gibson-Kueh S, Yang R, Thuy NTN, Jones JB, Nicholls PK, Ryan U. The molecular characterization of an Eimeria and Cryptosporidium detected in Asian seabass (Lates calcarifer) cultured in Vietnam. Veterinary Parasitology (Netherlands). 2011 Sep;**181**(2-4):91-96

[83] Yang R, Fenwick S, Potter A, Elliot A, Power M, Beveridge I, et al. Molecular characterization of Eimeria species in macropods. Experimental Parasitology (United States). 2012 Oct;**132**(2):216-221

[84] Chapman HD, Barta JR, Blake D, Gruber A, Jenkins M, Smith NC, et al. A selective review of advances in coccidiosis research. Advances in Parasitology (England). 2013;**83**:93-171

[85] Jirku M, Kvicerova J, Modry D, Hypsa V. Evolutionary plasticity in coccidia - striking morphological similarity of unrelated coccidia (apicomplexa) from related hosts: Eimeria spp. from African and Asian Pangolins (Mammalia: Pholidota). Protist (Germany). 2013 Jul;**164**(4):470-481

[86] Kvicerova J, Hypsa V. Host-parasite incongruences in rodent Eimeria suggest significant role of adaptation rather than cophylogeny in maintenance of host specificity. PLoS One (United States). 2013;**8**(7):e63601

[87] Blake DP. Eimeria genomics: Where are we now and where are we going? Veterinary Parasitology (Netherlands). 2015 Aug;**212**(1-2):68-74

[88] Long PL, Millard BJ, Joyner LP, Norton CC. A guide to laboratory techniques used in the study and diagnosis of avian coccidiosis. Folia Veterinaria Latina (Italy). 1976;**6**(3):201-217

[89] Revets H, Dekegel D, Deleersnijder W, De Jonckheere J, Peeters J, Leysen E, et al. Identification of virus-like particles in Eimeria stiedae. Molecular and Biochemical Parasitology (Netherlands). 1989 Oct;**36**(3):209-215

[90] Novilla MN, Carpenter JW. Pathology and pathogenesis of disseminated visceral coccidiosis in cranes. Avian Pathology (England). 2004 Jun;**33**(3):275-280

[91] Reid AJ, Blake DP, Ansari HR, Billington K, Browne HP, Bryant J, et al. Genomic analysis of the causative agents of coccidiosis in domestic chickens. Genome Research (United States). 2014 Oct;**24**(10):1676-1685

[92] Chapman HD, Shirley MW. The Houghton strain of Eimeria tenella: A review of the type strain selected for genome sequencing. Avian Pathology (England). 2003 Apr;**32**(2):115-127

[93] Shirley MW, Smith AL, Tomley FM. The biology of avian Eimeria with an emphasis on their control by vaccination. Advances in Parasitology (England). 2005;**60**:285-330

[94] Shirley MW, Harvey DA. A genetic linkage map of the apicomplexan protozoan parasite Eimeria tenella. Genome Research (United States). 2000 Oct;**10**(10):1587-1593

[95] Ling K-H, Rajandream M-A, Rivailler P, Ivens A, Yap S-J, Madeira AMBN, et al. Sequencing and analysis of chromosome 1 of Eimeria tenella reveals a unique segmental organization. Genome Research (United States). 2007 Mar;**17**(3):311-319

[96] Dubey JP, Carpenter JL, Speer CA, Topper MJ, Uggla A. Newly recognized fatal protozoan disease of dogs. Journal of the American Veterinary Medical Association (United States). 1988 May;**192**(9):1269-1285

[97] Dubey JP, Barr BC, Barta JR, Bjerkas I, Bjorkman C, Blagburn BL, et al. Redescription of Neospora caninum and its differentiation from related coccidia. International Journal for Parasitology (England). 2002 Jul;**32**(8):929-946

[98] McCann CM, Vyse AJ, Salmon RL, Thomas D, Williams DJL, McGarry JW, et al. Lack of serologic evidence of Neospora caninum in humans, England. Emerging Infectious Diseases (United States). 2008 Jun;**14**(6):978-980

[99] Dubey JP, Schares G, Ortega-Mora LM. Epidemiology and Control of Neosporosis and Neospora caninum. Clinical Microbiology Reviews. 2007;**20**:323-367

[100] Davison HC, Otter A, Trees AJ. Estimation of vertical and horizontal transmission parameters of Neospora caninum infections in dairy cattle. International Journal for Parasitology (England). 1999 Oct;**29**(10):1683-1689

[101] Trees AJ, Davison HC, Innes EA, Wastling JM. Towards evaluating the economic impact of bovine neosporosis. International Journal for Parasitology (England). 1999 Aug;**29**(8):1195-1200

[102] Reid AJ, Vermont SJ, Cotton JA, Harris D, Hill-Cawthorne GA, Konen-Waisman S, et al. Comparative genomics of the apicomplexan parasites Toxoplasma gondii and Neospora caninum: Coccidia differing in host range and transmission strategy. PLoS Pathogens (United States). 2012;**8**(3):e1002567

[103] Hornok S, Mester A, Takacs N, Baska F, Majoros G, Fok E, et al. Sarcocystis-infection of cattle in Hungary. Parasites & Vectors (England). 2015;**8**:69

[104] Blazejewski T, Nursimulu N, Pszenny V, Dangoudoubiyam S, Namasivayam S, Chiasson MA, et al. Systems-based analysis of the Sarcocystis neurona genome identifies pathways that contribute to a heteroxenous life cycle. MBio (United States). 2015;**6**(1)

[105] Cowper B, Matthews S, Tomley F. The molecular basis for the distinct host and tissue tropisms of coccidian parasites. Molecular and Biochemical Parasitology (Netherlands). 2012 Nov;**186**(1):1-10

[106] Dubey JP, Lindsay DS, Saville WJ, Reed SM, Granstrom DE, Speer CA. A review of Sarcocystis neurona and equine protozoal myeloencephalitis (EPM). Veterinary Parasitology (Netherlands). 2001 Feb;**95**(2-4):89-131

[107] Fayer R, Esposito DH, Dubey JP. Human infections with Sarcocystis species. Clinical Microbiology Reviews (United States). 2015 Apr;**28**(2):295-311

[108] Dubey JP, Lindsay DS. Neosporosis, toxoplasmosis, and sarcocystosis in ruminants. Veterinary Clinics of North America: Food Animal Practice. (United States). 2006 Nov;**22**(3):645-671

[109] More G, Pantchev A, Skuballa J, Langenmayer MC, Maksimov P, Conraths FJ, et al. Sarcocystis sinensis is the most prevalent thick-walled Sarcocystis species in beef on sale for consumers in Germany. Parasitology Research (Germany). 2014 Jun;**113**(6):2223-2230

[110] Dubey JP, Fayer R, Rosenthal BM, Calero-Bernal R, Uggla A. Identity of Sarcocystis species of the water buffalo (Bubalus bubalis) and cattle (Bos taurus) and the suppression of Sarcocystis sinensis as a nomen nudum. Veterinary Parasitology (Netherlands). 2014 Sep;**205**(1-2):1-6

[111] Chen X, Zuo Y, Rosenthal BM, He Y, Cui L, Yang Z. Sarcocystis sinensis is an ultrastructurally distinct parasite of water buffalo that can cause foodborne illness but cannot complete its life-cycle in human beings. Veterinary Parasitology (Netherlands). 2011 May;**178**(1-2):35-39

[112] Saito M, Shibata Y, Ohno A, Kubo M, Shimura K, Itagaki H. Sarcocystis suihominis detected for the first time from pigs in Japan. The Journal of Veterinary Medical Science (Japan). 1998 Mar;**60**(3):307-309

[113] Miller MA, Crosbie PR, Sverlow K, Hanni K, Barr BC, Kock N, et al. Isolation and characterization of Sarcocystis from brain tissue of a free-living southern sea otter (Enhydra lutris nereis) with fatal meningoencephalitis. Parasitology Research (Germany). 2001 Mar;**87**(3):252-257

Chapter 7

Avian Coccidiosis, New Strategies of Treatment

Rosa Estela Quiroz-Castañeda

Additional information is available at the end of the chapter

http://dx.doi.org/10.5772/intechopen.74008

Abstract

The control of avian coccidiosis since the 1940s has been associated with the use of ionophores and chemical drugs. Recently, a significant interest in natural sources has developed due to the pressure to poultry industry to produce drug-free birds. Consequently, the search of products derived from plants and other natural sources has increased in the last years. Today, many commercial products containing essential oils, extracts, and other compounds are available. The use of these compounds of natural origin is related to an increased immune response, a body weight gain, destruction of oocyst, among other benefits. The main inconvenience of these products is the act on some species of *Eimeria*, but not all. This genetic variability found in the parasite makes the use of products difficult to control and treat coccidiosis. In this chapter, several proposals of treatment are presented based on the use of natural products, considering the new strategies of treatment with minimal consequences to birds.

Keywords: *Eimeria*, coccidiosis, natural treatments, vaccines, herbal extracts

1. Introduction

Chickens' production is positioned as an important source of meat around the world. About 60 billion chickens are produced worldwide every year. However, *Eimeria* protozoan parasites of Phylum Apicomplexa are considered the main risk to avian production since they are the causative agent of avian coccidiosis [1]. For Avian coccidiosis is caused by seven species of *Eimeria*, which parasite chickens intestine resulting in economic losses around $2.4 billion per year worldwide [2].

The life cycle of the *Eimeria* is complex. They have developmental cycles with an exogenous phase in the environment and an endogenous phase in the intestine of chickens [3]. The efforts to prevent this disease have been focused on developing vaccines and drugs with coccidiostatic and coccidicidal activity [4]. So far, genomic studies have revealed the wide antigenic variability of species such as *Eimeria tenella,* one of the most pathogenic parasites to chickens, which leads to develop a vaccine resistance rapidly [1].

The main problem of coccidiosis treatment is that the resistance to anticoccidial drugs can evolve rapidly leading to a continuing need to develop novel and effective therapies [5].

In this chapter, avian coccidiosis is briefly reviewed and a special focus on novel strategies of treatment is presented. The strategies include the use of herbal compounds to genomic analysis of *Eimeria* species.

2. Avian coccidiosis

Poultry industry raises approximately 40 billion chickens annually and more than 100 tonnes of chicken meat. Today, there exist a growing demand of this meat not only because it is cheaper than other types of meat, but also due to the increasing number of inhabitants around the world [6]. In spite of the high production of poultry industry which still exists, some factors are affecting the productivity such as handling, housing, and rearing of birds in addition to disease control (nutritional, metabolic, and parasitic diseases) [7].

2.1. Causative agents of coccidiosis

Avian coccidiosis is a parasitic disease caused by protozoa belonging to the phylum Apicomplexa, genus *Eimeria.* It affects virtually all domestic and wild species, causing signs such as paleness, diarrhea with or without blood, high feed conversion, weight loss, and in severe cases even death. It is the most important parasitic disease of the poultry industry worldwide, causing serious economic losses both for the prevention and the control of subclinical or clinical disease [8]. The disease transmission is fecal-oral by consuming oocysts eliminated by infected birds. Those oocysts present in bed sporulate when conditions are favorable. Currently, the problem tends to worsen because conditions of intensive poultry production as the amount of oocysts per m^2 in bed are higher and therefore, the challenge for the birds [9].

More than 1200 species of *Eimeria* are described, most of them parasitizing the intestinal epithelium of vertebrates, and as a consequence, infected birds reduce feed intake, have bloody diarrhea, and have hampered weight gains [10].

In domestic fowl (*Gallus gallus domesticus*), seven species of *Eimeria* are reported. Those causing hemorrhagic disease are *E. brunetti, E. necatrix,* and *E. tenella.* Considered as mildly pathogenic and causing malabsorptive disease *E. acervulina, E. mitis, E, maxima,* and *E. praecox* [5]. Each species has a specific site of development in the small intestine (upper, middle, lower, rectum, and caeca) **Table 1**.

2.2. Life cycle

Eimeria life cycle is complex and comprises of three stages, one occurs on litter under the conditions of humidity, temperature, and oxygen supply (sporogony), and two stages occurs in

http://dx.doi.org/10.5772/intechopen.74008

Species	Site of development	Pathogenicity	Disease type
E. necatrix	Jejunum, ileum, caeca	+++++	Hemorrhagic
E. brunetti	Caeca and rectum	++++	Hemorrhagic
E. tenella	Caeca	++++	Hemorrhagic
E. maxima	Jejunum, ileum	+++	Malabsorptive
E. mitis	Ileum	++	Malabsorptive
E. acervulina	Duodenum, ileum	++	Malabsorptive
E. praecox	Duodenum, jejunum	+	Malabsorptive

Table 1. Location and pathogenicity of ***Eimeria*** species [5, 7].

the cells of intestinal epithelium [merogony or schizogony (asexual reproduction) and gametogony (sexual reproduction)].

During the sporogony, which is considered a noninfective stage, the oocyst is excreted in chicken feces and undergoes sporulation in the presence of humidity, warmth, and oxygen and thus becoming a sporulated oocyst, now infective. Merogony or schizogony occurs in the intestine and comprises of several rounds of asexual multiple division (from two to four times), followed by gametogony that involves the formation of male and female gametes, fertilization and formation of a zygote (oocyst) that will be excreted in feces [11]. Infection starts when the host ingest sporulated oocysts (**Figure 1**).

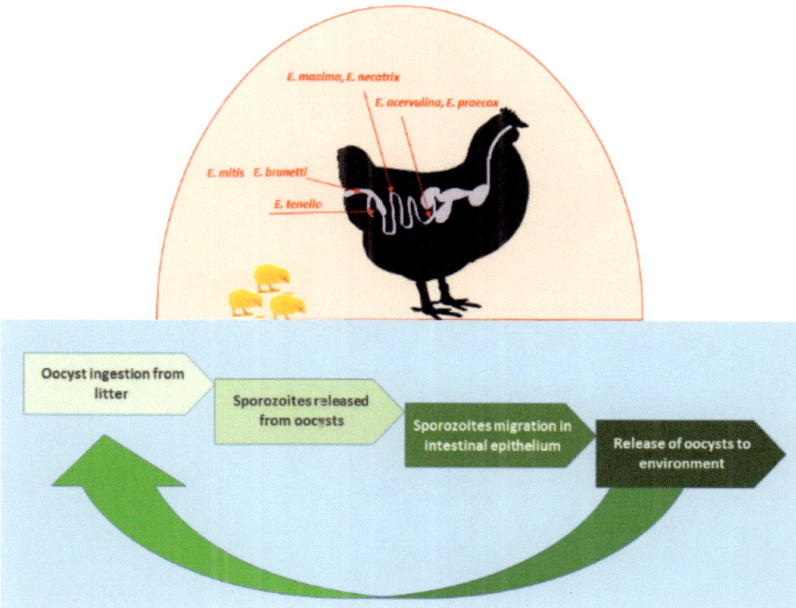

Figure 1. Infection process of *Eimeria* spp. in chickens. First, *Eimeria* oocysts are ingested by chickens, once inside, *Eimeria* sporozoites colonize and infect different regions of intestine epithelium. Oocysts are formed again and released to litter to begin another cycle.

Due to the chemical and mechanical proventriculus and gizzard action, and the presence of CO_2 in the lumen, the oocyst releases the sporozoites, which gets the intestinal lumen and attached to enterocytes using this anchoring and penetration proteins present in the apical complex (rhoptries and micronemes) entering the cell in order to continue the second phase: esquizogony or merogony, producing a schizont with thousands of merozoites inside to be released back into the lumen to infect new intestinal cells. Thus, after several stages of merogonies, some of the merozoites inside the intestinal cell forms macrogamonts with a macrogametocyte (inmobile cell considered the female gamete) and some forms microgamonts with several microgametocytes inside (mobile cells considered male gametes). These microgametocytes come out of the cells that originated to locate and fertilize to macrogametocyte producing a zygote to be excreted in the feces again (not sporulated oocyst) to begin another cycle [12] **Figure 2**.

Once the oocyst is formed, it is considered the most persistent structure of *Eimeria* life cycle. It has a significant resistance to mechanical, chemical, and proteolytic damage, due to the composition of the two walls that confer the oocyst and outstanding resistance [13, 14] **Figure 3**.

The unsporulated oocyst is considered as the noninfective stage while the sporulated oocyst is the infective stage, in *Eimeria,* the oocyst has four sporocysts, each with two sporozoites **Figure 4**.

Environmental factors such as humidity (40–80%), temperature (24–28°C), and oxygen supply (aeration) makes the sporulation occurs, at least in *E. acervulina* the most important environmental

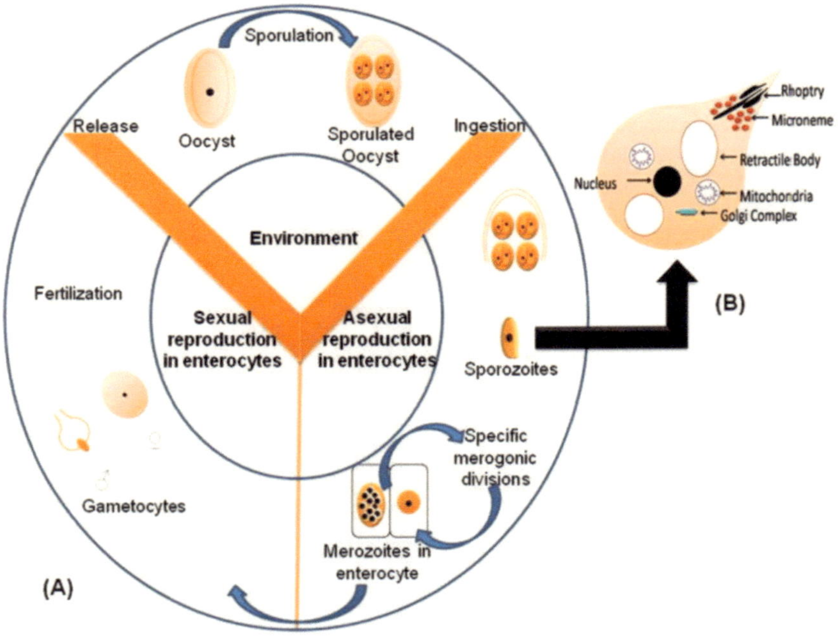

Figure 2. Life cycle of *Eimeria*. (A) Sexual and asexual stages reproduction occurs in epithelium cells and oocyst formation occurs outside the birds under specific environmental conditions. (B) Structure of *Eimeria* spp. sporozoite. Figure taken from https://doi.org/10.1016/j.trivac.2016.02.001.

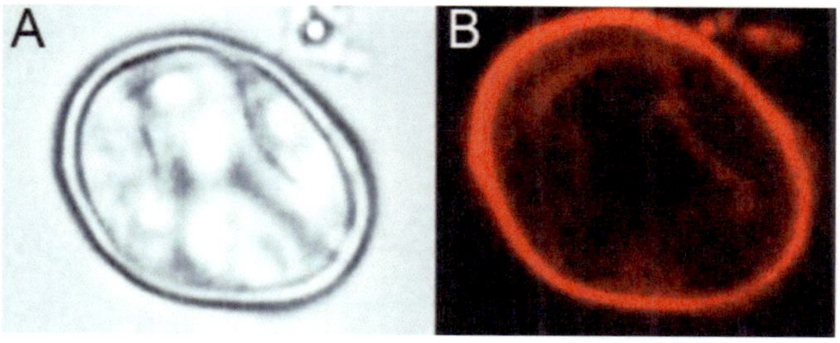

Figure 3. *Eimeria* oocyst cell wall micrograph. Double layer of oocyst is observed. (A) Bright-field of *Eimeria* oocyst and (B) Oocyst staining with FM™ 4-64FX fluorophore. M. A. Castelló-Leyva. Faculty of Veterinary and Animal Sciences, UNAM.

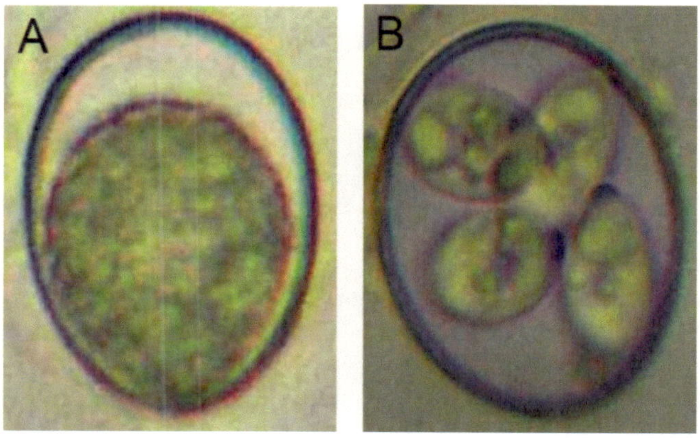

Figure 4. *Eimeria* oocyst bright-field micrograph. (A) Unsporulated oocyst. (B) Sporulated oocyst, the infective stage, containing four sporocysts. Notice the double layer of cell wall. M. A. Castelló-Leyva. Faculty of Veterinary and Animal Sciences, UNAM.

factor to onset sporulation is temperature [15, 16]. Nevertheless, the temperature is an environmental factor that is hard to control due to the ideal temperatures that are easily reached in the poultry litter.

3. Strategies of treatment

During the last years, research has focused on development of anticoccidial drugs, with interest focused on the sexual and asexual stages of the parasites (stages occurring within the host). However, exists a tendency to ban the use of drugs in animals for human consumption, so the development of new drugs to control avian coccidiosis demands another way to control the disease.

The control of avian coccidiosis is a challenge of veterinary parasitology. So far, any treatment, including, anticoccidial drugs, vaccines, or natural alternatives control avian coccidiosis by itself. It proposed the use of combination of different strategies to achieve an effective control (**Figure 5**).

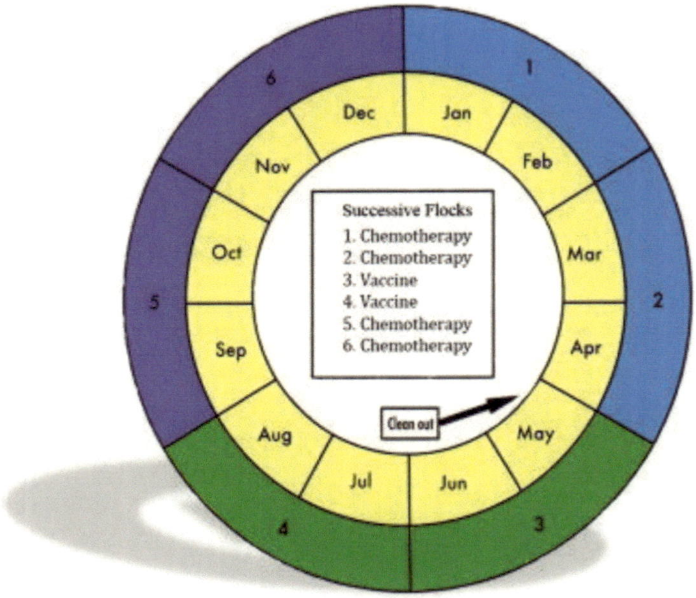

Figure 5. The proposal of use of chemotherapy and vaccines in a yearly chicken production. Figure taken from [17]. In the clean out period litter is removed. Chemotherapy comprises use of anticoccidial drugs.

3.1. Chemotherapy

This treatment comprises of ionophorous compounds (ionophores) and synthetic drugs (chemicals). Ionophores usually cause the death of parasite and are produced by the fermentation and chemicals inhibit several biochemical pathways of the parasite and are produced by chemical synthesis [17, 18]. In **Table 2**, the most important ionophores and chemicals are shown.

Treatment	Examples	Function
Ionophores	Lasalocid, Monensin, Narasinm Salinomycin, and Semduramicin	Disruption of ion gradient across the parasite cell membrane
Chemicals	Quinolone drugs (Decoquinate and nequinatem buquinolate).	Inhibition of parasite mitochondrial respiration
	Pyridones (Meticlorpindol)	
	Sulphonamides	Inhibition of the folic acid pathway
	Amprolium	Competitive inhibition of thiamine uptake
	Diclazuril, Halofuginone, and Robenidine	Mode of action unknown
	Nicarbazin	Inhibition of the development of the first and second generations of the schizont stage of the parasites

Table 2. Most commonly used ionophores and chemical in coccidiosis treatment.

However, after prolonged uses of a drug treatment, several drug-resistant strains may emerge, which represents a severe problem [19]. To combat resistance, shuttle, mix, and rotation systems of drugs are employed.

3.2. Vaccines

Passive or active immune responses induce immunity in animals. This immunity can reduce the pathogenic effects of coccidiosis such as less macroscopically visible lesions, decreasing of oocyst production, and increasing performance of birds [16].

The first commercial live coccidiosis vaccine was CocciVac® registered in the USA in 1952 [20]. Currently, two types of vaccines are used with the aim of controlling coccidiosis in a chemical-free way: nonattenuated and attenuated vaccines.

The main risk of using live nonattenuated vaccines (Coccivac, Advent, Immucox, and Inovocox) is the live parasites that can develop a severe reaction in birds. Many times their use is accompanied by chemical treatments to control the inherent pathogenicity of the parasites [21].

On the contrary, the success of live attenuated vaccines (Paracox and HatchPak CocciIII) relies on the low risk of disease occurring because of the reduction in the proliferation of parasites and consequently a less damage in birds' tissue [22].

Nonattenuated and attenuated vaccines may have different routes of administration (oral, eyes drops, in ovo) in birds and several *Eimeria* species as target [23].

Subunit vaccines consist of purified antigenic determinants obtained from *Eimeria* parasite. These vaccines are obtained from DNA recombinant technology and may consist of native antigens or recombinant proteins of various stages (sporozoites, merozoites, and gametes) of *Eimeria* [16]. Distinct protective antigens used are micronemes, rhoptries, refractile bodies, merozoites, or gametocytes of *Eimeria* parasite [24].

These kinds of vaccines involve native or recombinant subunit second generation extract or DNA vaccines. The only commercial subunit vaccine was CoxAbic®, based on purified native protein isolated from gametocytes of *Eimeria* and inhibits the development of oocysts but with only 53% of protection against challenge with *Eimeria* infections, resulting in a very limiting vaccine [22, 25].

Proteomic analysis of *E. tenella* life cycle stages (unsporulated oocyst, sporulated oocyst, sporozoite, and second generation merozoite) revealed specific proteins in each stage and many other proteins are shared in all stages. During parasite invasion, proteins RON2 and RON5 are expressed, these proteins have been previously identified in *Toxoplasma gondii,* and also were found in *E. tenella*, where may have a role in host adhesion during process of invasion [11].

A collection of epitope mapping of T-cell mediated antigenic determinants was applied in an *in silico* analysis to investigate promising epitopes from the sporozoite and merozoite stages. Several epitopes showed a significant predicted efficacy [26].

So far, the use of recombinant vaccines is limited mainly due to the low protection of antigens with the potential to induce potent protective immune response against *Eimeria*. Certainly, genomic and proteomic analyses of *E. tenella* genome will allow the design and development of potential immunogens that could be used as vaccine in future [5, 27, 28].

3.3. Natural compounds, alternative treatments

The search of alternatives to anticoccidial drugs and vaccines against avian coccidiosis has led to discover in fungal extracts, plant extracts, and probiotics a source of new compounds with anticoccidial activity. Many of them with the oocyst as target being that if the dispersion of oocysts is controlled then the possibilities of infection reduce.

The role of fats, essential oils and herbal and medicinal plants has been explored to control avian coccidiosis.

3.3.1. Fats

Fatty acids from fish or flax seeds reduce the severity of *E. tenella* infections in young broiler chicks. Diets supplemented with docosahexaenoic acid, linoleic acid, and eicosapentaenoic acid allowed a maintained weight gain in birds, which strongly suggests their use as part or birds nutrition. Cecal lesions were reduced as well as the parasite invasion rate and development of parasite. Unfortunately, this benefits only were observed in birds infected with *E. tenella* and not with other species, thus, limiting the use of fatty acids to control coccidiosis [29, 30].

3.3.2. Essential oils

The use of essential oils as a therapy to control *Eimeria* oocysts is widely reported. Although the mechanism of oils is still unclear, they destroy the most resistant structure of *Eimeria*, the oocyst, thus reducing dispersion and the risk of infection [7].

Functional oils comprise those oils that have an action beyond nutritional value [31]. Recently, a variety of essential have been used at different stages of life cycle of *Eimeria* with good results **Figure 6**.

In vitro assays are used to test potential oocysticidal activity of essential oils. The use of oils from Artemisia, thyme, tea tree, and clove showed a clear destruction of oocyst after 3 hours of treatment and a $LC_{50} < 1$ mg/ml of oocyst [33]. Commercial oils carvacol, carvone, isopulegol, thymol, and eugenol were used to destroy a mixture of *Eimeria* species oocysts, a release of oocyst internal substances was observed after treatment suggesting the potential of these oils to control oocysts of *E. tenella, E. maxima, E. acervulina, E. necatrix,* and *E. mitis* [34].

A commercial essential oils product called Essential (Oligo Basics Agroind. Ltda, www.oligobasics.com.br) containing ricinoleic acid and alkylphenolic oil of the shell of the cashew nut (*Anacardium occidentale*) showed an improvement in the energy utilization and the livability and decreased lesion caused by coccidiosis (*E. acervulina, E.maxima,* and *E. tenella*) in birds treated with Essential [31].

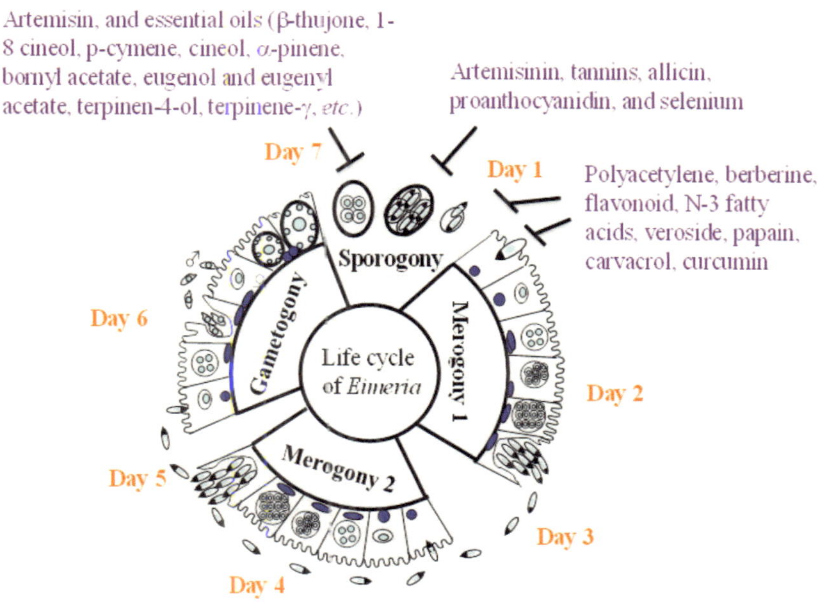

Figure 6. Plant compounds target different stages of life cycle of *Eimeria* species. Different phytocompounds inhibit the sporogony and merogony stages. Figure reproduced with permission from [32].

3.3.3. Herbal derivatives

A total of 68 plants and phytocompounds with proven suppression of *Eimeria* species have been reported. Some plants species and their extracted compounds with anticoccidial effects are: Fabacea: *Sophora flavescens, Gleditsia japonica;* Menispermaceae: *Sinomenium acutum;* Combretaceae: *Quisqualis indica;* Ranunculaceae, *Pulsatilla koreana;* Ulmaceae: *Ulmus macrocarpa;* Asteraceae: *Artemisia asiatica, Artemisia sieberi, Artemisia afra;* Meliaceae: *Melia azedarach;* Piperaceae: *Piper nigrum* Urticaceae: *Urtica dioica;* Brassicaceae: *Lepidium sativum,* Apiaceae: *Foeniculum vulgare;* Rubiaceae: *Morinda lucida;* Burseraceae: *Commiphora swynnertonii,* Moringaceae: *Moringa oleifera, Moringa indica, Moringa stenopetala;* Lamiaceae: *Origanum* spp., *Lavandula stoechas; Mentha arvensis;* Lauraceae: *Laurus nobilis;* Musaceae: *Musa paradisiaca;* Solanaceae: *Solanum nigrum;* Meliaceae: *Melia azadirachta;* Amaryllidaceae: *Tulbaghia violacea,* Vitaceae: *Vitis vinifera;* Fagaceae: *Quercus infectoria;* Anacardiaceae: *Rhus chinensis* and Combretaceae: *Terminalia chebula* [32].

The usage of these plants varies from organic extracts (ethanol, petroleum ether and acetone extracts), ground powder, essential oils, and decoction. The parameters measured to evaluate efficiency of the anticoccidial compounds are body weight gain, oocyst count, feed consumption, lesion scores, bloody diarrhea, and mortality [7, 32]. Recently, plant *Bidens pilosa* was used in diet of birds, which significantly elevated body weight gain and lowered feed conversion ratio. Also, *B. pilosa* reduced cecal damage, villus destruction and decreased villus-to-crypt ratio in chicken ceca [35, 36].

Table 3 shows some compounds related to different action to control avian coccidiosis. Information based on [7, 32, 37].

The use of these compounds is not limited to laboratory conditions, many products that contain natural compounds are commercially available for prevention and treatment of coccidiosis. This highlights their potential use in poultry industry. In **Table 4**, commercial natural products are show.

Action	Compound (Plant/fungi)	Function
Inhibition of *Eimeria* life cycle	Artemisin (*Artemisia annua*)	Induce reactive oxygen species (ROS) that inhibit oocyst wall formation and sporulation
	Tannins, Pine (*Pinus radiata*)	Inhibition of life cycle and decreased sporulation of the oocyst
	Allicin and sulfur compounds, Garlic (*Allium sativum*)	Antimicrobial activity and inhibition of sporulation of *E. tenella*.
	Selenium, Phenolics and Green tea (*Camellia sinensis)*	Inhibition of sporulation of coccidian oocysts.
	Papain (*Carica papaya)*	Inhibition of coccidiosis probably by proteolytic degradation of *Eimeria*
	Saponins (*Cyamopsis tetragonoloba)*	Suppression of coccidiosis
	Essential oils from thyme, tea tree and clove	Destruction of *Eimeria* oocysts
	Ethyl acetate extract (*Meyerozyma guilliermondii*)	Destruction of *Eimeria* spp. oocysts
Immune response modulators	Probiotics (*Pediococcus acidilactici* and *Saccharomyces boulardii*)	Enhanced humoral immunity, changes in body weight gain and fecal oocyst shedding rates.
	Arabinoxylans (*Triticum aestivum*) Sugar cane (*Saccharum officinarum*)	Immunostimulatory and protective effects against coccidiosis in broiler chickens
	Polysaccharides (*Astragalus membranaceus Radix, Carthamus tinctorius, Lentinula edodes, Tremella fuciformis)*	Enhancement of anticoccidial antibodies and antigen-specific cell proliferation in splenocytes via cellular and humoral immunity to *E. tenella*
	Phytonutrients mixtures: VAC (carvacrol, cinnamaldehyde, *Capsicum* oleoresin). MC (*Capsicum* oleoresin and turmeric oleoresin)	Protection against *E. tenella* infection. Increase in NK cells, macrophages, CD4+ T cells, CD8 + T cells and cytokines IFN γ and IL6.
	Lectins (*Fomitella fraxinea*)	Enhancement of both cellular and humoral immune response

Table 3. Natural compounds identified with potential to inhibit ***Eimeria*** life cycle and acting as immune system modulators.

Commercial name	Ingredients	Producer
Essential	Ricinoleic acid and alkylphenolic oil of the shell of the cashew nut (*Anacardium occidentale*)	Oligo Basics Agroind. Ltda,
Avihicox	Clove and *Bocconia cordata* extract	Centaur
Nutrimin	Apple cider vinegar	Chicken Lickin
Kochi free	Olive leaf, mustard seed, black seed, cloves, grapefruit seed extract	Amber Technology
Coccinon	Blend of plant extracts and natural compounds	Natural farm health
Oil of oregano	80% Carvacrol	Natural factors
Garlic granules	Garlic	Flyte so fancy
Poultry Provita	Probiotics and prebiotic inulin	Vets plus
Eimericox	Blend of essential oils	Phytosynthese/Trouw nutrition
Enteroguard	Garlic and cinnamon	Orffa
Coxynil	*Allium sativum* Linn 15%, *Cinnamomum camphora* Nees & Eberum 15%, *Elephantopus scaber* Linn 15%, *Valeriana wallichii* DC 15%, Sulfur dioxide 25% and NaCl 15%	Growell India

Table 4. Commercially available compounds of natural origin: plants and herbal extracts, fatty acids, probiotics and others).

4. Future vision of avian coccidiosis

The development of new treatments against avian coccidiosis is a challenge to many researchers. However, information of parasites still can be revealed using new strategies such as omics approaches. Recently, a transcriptional profile analysis of virulent and precocious strains of *E. tenella* revealed that some genes involved in carbohydrate metabolism, proteases, transporters, cell attachment proteins, and mitochondrial proteins express are upregulated in the virulent strain [38].

The vaccine development against *Eimeria* spp. also requires new approaches. Marugan-Hernández et al., [39] reported the expression of viral proteins in parasite *E. tenella*. They found that the chicken immune system recognizes the expressed viral proteins, which is a significant precedent to develop a vaccine in future, due to the chance to express antigens that allow recognition of the parasite. A study about the population structure or *E. tenella* as well as their genotype distribution and the presence of the Apical Membrane Antigen 1 (AMA1) showed that this antigen outweighs immune evasion [1].

The recent studies of *Eimeria* spp. focus on genomic, transcriptomic, and proteomic analysis, besides genetic diversity and molecular phylogenetics, which strengthens the need to explore other fields of interest [5, 40–42].

5. Conclusions

The development of drugs to control and treat avian coccidiosis since the 1940s until now has increased significantly leading to a wide variety of products. The use of these drugs interferes with cofactor synthesis, mitochondrial functions, and cell membrane function of *Eimeria* spp. Although their use was the first alternative, today, most governments and health policies preferred meal free of antibiotics and drugs, as in most European countries.

This view guided research efforts to search for new compounds with a natural origin. Thus, plants, fungi, and bacteria were considered sources of metabolites and molecules with potential anticoccidial activity. In this chapter, we present recent information related to compounds that can be used to prevent, control, and treat avian coccidiosis. Many of them were with good results when an immune response is involved.

This disease may not be controlled or treated with the use of only one compound, on the contrary, it requires the combination of immunostimulators that induce a good response in bird and herbal extracts, essential oils and other natural compounds that can destroy *Eimeria* spp. oocysts or interfere with life cycle. In summary, avian coccidiosis control demands many shared efforts that with the advancement of omics technologies will certainly open new lines of investigation.

Author details

Rosa Estela Quiroz-Castañeda

Address all correspondence to: quiroz.rosa@inifap.gob.mx

Anaplasmosis Unit, National Center for Disciplinary Research in Veterinary Parasitology, CENID-PAVET, INIFAP, Jiutepec, Morelos, México

References

[1] Blake DP, Clark EL, Macdonald SE, Thenmozhi V, Kundu K, Garg R, et al. Population, genetic, and antigenic diversity of the apicomplexan *Eimeria tenella* and their relevance to vaccine development. Proceedings of the National Academy of Sciences of the United States of America [Internet]. 2015;**112**(38):E5343-E5350. Available from: http://www.pubmedcentral.nih.gov/articlerender.fcgi?artid=4586875&tool=pmcentrez&rendertype=abstract

[2] Shirley MW, Smith AL, Tomley FM. The biology of avian Eimeria with an emphasis on their control by vaccination. Advances in Parasitology. 2005;**60**:285-330

[3] Lal K, Bromley E, Oakes R, Prieto JH, Sanya J, Kurian D, et al. Proteomic comparison of four Eimeria tenella life cycle stages. Proteomics. 2010;**9**(19):4566-4476

[4] Tewari AK, Maharana BR. Control of poultry coccidiosis: Changing trends. Journal of Parasitic Diseases. 2011;**35**(1):10-17

[5] Reid AJ, Blake DP, Ansari HR, Billington K, Browne HP, Bryant J, et al. Genomic analysis of the causative agents of coccidiosis in domestic chickens. Genome Research. 2014 Oct;**24**(10):1676-1685

[6] Faostat. FAOSTAT [Internet]. Livestock Primary. 2014. Available from: http://www.fao.org

[7] Quiroz-Castañeda RE, Dantán-González E. Control of avian coccidiosis: Future and present natural alternatives. BioMed Research International. 2015;**2015**:11. Article ID: 430610. http://dx.doi.org/10.1155/2015/430610

[8] Chapman HD, Barta JR, Blake D, Gruber A, Jenkins M, Smith NC, et al. A selective review of advances in coccidiosis research. Advances in Parasitology. 2013;**83**:93-171

[9] Haug A, Gjevre AG, Thebo P, Mattsson JG, Kaldhusdal M. Coccidial infections in commercial broilers: epidemiological aspects and comparison of Eimeria species identification by morphometric and polymerase chain reaction techniques. Avian Pathology [Internet]. 2008;**37**:161-170. Available from: http://dx.doi.org/10.1080/03079450801915130

[10] Gilbert ER, Cox CM, Williams PM, McElroy AP, Dalloul RA, Ray WK, et al. Eimeria species and genetic background influence the serum protein profile of broilers with coccidiosis. PLoS One [Internet]. 2011;**6**(1):e14636. Available from: http://dx.doi.org/10.1371/journal.pone.0014636

[11] Lal K, Bromley E, Oakes R, Prieto JH, Sanderson SJ, Kurian D, et al. Proteomic comparison of four Eimeria tenella life cycle stages: unsporulated oocyst, sporulated oocyst, sporozoite and second generation merozoite. Proteomics [Internet]. 2009;**9**(19):4566-4576. Available from: http://dx.doi.org/10.1002/pmic.200900305

[12] The Poultry Site. Coccidiosis Management for Natural and Organic Poultry [Internet]. 2017. Available from: http://www.thepoultrysite.com/publications/2/CoccidiosisManagement/41/life-cycle-and-types-of-coccidia/

[13] Belli SI, Smith NC, Ferguson DJ. The coccidian oocyst: A tough nut to crack! Trends in Parasitology [Internet]. 2006;**22**(9):4169-4423. Available from: http://dx.doi.org/10.1016/j.pt.2006.07.004

[14] Mai K, Sharman PA, Walker RA, Katrib M, Souza D, McConville MJ, et al. Oocyst wall formation and composition in coccidian parasites. Memórias do Instituto Oswaldo Cruz [Internet]. 2009;**104**(2):281-289. Available from: http://dx.doi.org/10.1590/S0074-02762009000200022

[15] Graat EAM, Henken AM, Ploeger HW, Noordhuizen JPTM, Vertommen MH. Rate and course of sporulation of oocysts of Eimeria acervulina under different environmental conditions. Parasitology [Internet]. 2009/04/01. 1994;**108**(5):497-502. Available from: https://www.cambridge.org/core/article/rate-and-course-of-sporulation-of-oocysts-of-eimeria-acervulina-under-different-environmental-conditions/90410949EA40127F9CEDE211C4370C60

[16] Peek HW, Landman WJM. Coccidiosis in poultry: Anticoccidial products, vaccines and other prevention strategies. The Veterinary Quarterly. 2011;**31**(3):143-161

[17] Chapman HD, Jeffers TK. Vaccination of chickens against coccidiosis ameliorates drug resistance in commercial poultry production. International Journal for Parasitology: Drugs and Drug Resistance [Internet]. 2014 Dec 25;**4**(3):214-217. Available from: http://www.ncbi.nlm.nih.gov/pmc/articles/PMC4266793/

[18] Chapman HD, Jeffers TK, Williams RB. Forty years of monensin for the control of coccidiosis in poultry. Poultry Science [Internet]. 2010;**89**(9):1788-1801. Available from: http://dx.doi.org/10.3382/ps.2010-00931

[19] McDougald LR. Protozoal infections. In: Saif YM, Barnes HJ, Glisson JR, Fadly AM, McDougald LR, Swayne DE, editors. Diseases of Poultry. Ames, IA, USA: Iowa State University Press; 2003. pp. 973-1023

[20] Edgar SA, King D. Breeding and immunizing chickens for resistance to coccidiosis 62nd and 63rd Annual Alabama Agricultural Experiment Station. 1952;36-37

[21] Williams S. Fifty years of anticoccidial vaccines for poultry (1952-2002). Avian Diseases. 2002;**46**(4):775-802

[22] Sharman PS, Smith SC, Wallach MG, Chasing KM. The golden egg: Vaccination against poultry coccidiosis. Parasite Immunology. 2010;**32**(8):590-598

[23] Williams RB. Anticoccidial vaccines for broiler chickens: Pathways to success. Avian Pathology [Internet]. 2002 Aug 1;**31**(4):317-353. Available from: http://dx.doi.org/10.1080/03079450220148988

[24] Jenkins MC. Advances and prospects for subunit vaccines against protozoa of veterinary importance. Veterinary Parasitology [Internet]. 2001 Nov 22;**101**(3-4):291-310. Available from: http://www.sciencedirect.com/science/article/pii/S030440170100557X

[25] Wallach M, Smith NC, Petracca M, Miller CMD, Eckert J, Braun R. Eimeria maxima gametocyte antigens: Potential use in a subunit maternal vaccine against coccidiosis in chickens. Vaccine [Internet]. 1995;**13**(4):347-354. Available from: http://www.sciencedirect.com/science/article/pii/0264410X95982559

[26] Ahmad TA, Tawfik DM, Sheweita SA, Haroun M, El-Sayed LH. Development of immunization trials against *Acinetobacter baumannii*. Trials in Vaccinology [Internet]. 2016;**5**:53-60. Available from: http://dx.doi.org/10.1016/j.trivac.2016.02.001

[27] Viljoen GJ, Luckins AG. The role of nuclear technologies in the diagnosis and control of livestock diseases–A review. Tropical Animal Health and Production. 2012;**44**(7):1341-1366

[28] Ling K-H, Rajandream M-A, Rivailler P, Ivens A, Yap S-J, Madeira AMBN, et al. Sequencing and analysis of chromosome 1 of *Eimeria tenella* reveals a unique segmental organization. Genome Research. 2007 Mar;**17**(3):311-319

[29] Allen PC, Danforth H, Levander OA. Interaction of dietary flaxseed with coccidia infections in chickens. Poultry Science. 1997 Jun;**76**(6):822-827

[30] Allen PC, Danforth HD, Levander OA. Diets high in n-3 fatty acids reduce cecal lesion scores in chickens infected with *Eimeria tenella*. Poultry Science. 1996 Feb;**75**(2):179-185

[31] Murakami AE, Eyng C, Torrent J. Effects of functional oils on coccidiosis and apparent metabolizable energy in broiler chickens. Asian Australasian Journal of Animal Sciences. 2014;**27**(7):981-989

[32] Muthamilselvan T, Kuo TF, Wu YC, Yang WC. Herbal remedies for coccidiosis control: A review of plants, compounds, and anticoccidial actions. Evidence-Based Complementary and Alternative Medicine. 2016;**2016**. Article ID: 2657981, 19 pages. http://dx.doi.org/10.1155/2016/2657981

[33] Remmal A, Achahbar S, Bouddine L, Chami N, Chami F. In vitro destruction of Eimeria oocysts by essential oils. Veterinary Parasitology [Internet]. 2011;**182**(2-4):121-126. Available from: http://dx.doi.org/10.1016/j.vetpar.2011.06.002

[34] Remmal A, Achahbar S, Bouddine L, Chami F, Chami N. Oocysticidal effect of essential oil components against chicken Eimeria oocysts. International Journal of Veterinary Sciences and Medicine. 2013;**2013**. Article ID: 599816, 8 pages. DOI: 10.5171/2013.599816

[35] Chang CLT, Chung CY, Kuo CH, Kuo TF, Yang CW, Yang WC. Beneficial effect of *Bidens pilosa* on body weight gain, food conversion ratio, gut bacteria and coccidiosis in chickens. PLoS One. 2016;**11**(1):e0146141. https://doi.org/10.1371/journal.pone.0146141

[36] Yang WC, Tien YJ, Chung CY, Chen YC, Chiou WH, Hsu SY, et al. Effect of *Bidens pilosa* on infection and drug resistance of Eimeria in chickens. Research in Veterinary Science [Internet]. 2015;**98**:74-81. Available from: http://dx.doi.org/10.1016/j.rvsc.2014.11.002

[37] Dantán-González E, Quiroz-Castañeda RE, Cobaxin-Cárdenas M, Valle-Hernández J, Gama-Mart'inez Y, Tinoco-Valencia JR, et al. Impact of *Meyerozyma guilliermondii* isolated from chickens against Eimeria sp. protozoan, an in vitro analysis. BMC Veterinary Research [Internet]. 2015;**11**(1):1-11. Available from: http://dx.doi.org/10.1186/s12917-015-0589-0

[38] Matsubayashi M, Kawahara F, Hatta T, Yamagishi J, Miyoshi T, Anisuzzaman, et al. Transcriptional profiles of virulent and precocious strains of *Eimeria tenella* at sporozoite stage; novel biological insight into attenuated asexual development. Infection, Genetics and Evolution. 2016 Jun;**40**:54-62

[39] Marugan-Hernandez V, Cockle C, Macdonald S, Pegg E, Crouch C, Blake DP, et al. Viral proteins expressed in the protozoan parasite *Eimeria tenella* are detected by the chicken immune system. Parasites & Vectors. 2016 Aug;**9**:463

[40] Blake DP. Eimeria Genomics: Where are we now and where are we going? Veterinary Parasitology. 2015 Aug;**212**(1-2):68-74

[41] Zhang Z, Wang S, Huang J, Liu L, Lu M, Li M, et al. Proteomic analysis of *Eimeria acervulina* sporozoite proteins interaction with duodenal epithelial cells by shotgun LC-MS/MS. Molecular and Biochemical Parasitology. 2015 Aug;**202**(2):29-33

[42] Kumar S, Garg R, Banerjee PS, Ram H, Kundu K, Kumar S, et al. Genetic diversity within ITS-1 region of Eimeria species infecting chickens of north India. Infection, Genetics and Evolution. 2015 Dec;**36**:262-267

Chapter 8

Natural Compounds as an Alternative to Control Farm Diseases: Avian Coccidiosis

Mayra E. Cobaxin-Cárdenas

Additional information is available at the end of the chapter

http://dx.doi.org/10.5772/intechopen.72638

Abstract

Coccidiosis is one of the most aggressive and expensive parasite diseases in poultry industry worldwide. Currently, the most used control techniques are chemoprophylaxis and anticoccidial feed additives. Although there is a great variety of commercial anticoccidial drugs and vaccines in the market, there is also a significant resistance to use them in animals with human as final consumer. To date, none available product offers effective protection toward coccidiosis; however, the search for novel strategies to control this disease continues, and natural products have arisen as a potential way to cope with avian coccidiosis. In this chapter, we highlight recent advances in natural compounds, their anticoccidial properties, and mechanisms.

Keywords: chickens, coccidiosis, *Eimeria*, anticoccidial, natural products

1. Introduction

Chicken is considered an animal food with high consumption around the world; so, the development of novel drugs and vaccines to cope with poultry diseases is essential for worldwide food safety. Today, investment on poultry research is focused on development of anticoccidial treatments that can control pathogens at different stages of growth. Avian coccidiosis is an intestinal disease caused by apicomplexan protozoa belonging to genus *Eimeria* and is considered the most economical important parasitic disease affecting poultry industry globally [1–3].

The study of *Eimeria* spp. has driven the search of new chemical or natural compounds in order to control infections, which may be caused by even more than one species that infect different regions of the chicken intestine. In addition, some other environmental and non-environmental factors can contribute to dispersion of *Eimeria* oocysts, such as *Eimeria* virulence, high oocyst challenge, poor ventilation, high stocking density, low immune status of the host, bacterial enteritis, high moisture levels in litters humidity and lower efficacy of anticoccidial drugs [4, 5].

Disease control includes vaccines, anticoccidial chemicals, coccidiostats, ionophores, probiotics, natural extracts, and natural compounds. However, the constant use of antibiotics induces selection of multidrug-resistant strains of parasites, besides the fact that drug residues may remain in poultry products for human consumption. This is why animal health regulations were established; for example, in European countries, prophylactic control based on mixtures of food with anticoccidial additives has been strongly limited since 2006 and they withdraw from the market in 2021 (Council Directive of 2011/50/EU of the European Council) [3, 6].

To cope with this situation, vaccination is the only preventive method that may help to control avian coccidiosis. In this regard, the use of natural compounds may be considered as an effective way to control coccidiosis in combination with integrated pest management. Research of natural products and the use of derivatives of plants have potential since these new therapeutic molecules are unknown to *Eimeria* strains and therefore they have not yet developed resistance [7]. The natural products used to control avian coccidiosis include plants [4], prebiotics, probiotics [4, 8], and fungi [9, 10].

2. Coccidiosis in poultry industry

Commercial poultry farming is expanding daily, and poultry is the most efficient source of animal-derived protein [11]. Chicken meat is considered as an important source of animal proteins and fats, as well as a source of a whole range of organic and inorganic substances [12].

Worldwide, poultry generation has tripled in the last two decades, and the world's chicken herd is close to 21 billion, but annual production of new individuals is more than 60 billion and delivers more than 1.1 trillion eggs and more than 90 million tons of meat [13].

Chicken meat production is growing rapidly around the world, with a significant increase in the production. In a short period, between 2000 and 2012, the global chicken meat market increased more than 58.48%. Fifty years ago, 79% of the chicken market was absorbed for American and European countries, but currently, Asian and American countries contributed approximately 77% of total world production according to reports in 2014 [4, 14]. Differential growth in production has been observed according to geographical location as follows: The Asian's production had the largest increase with more than 68.83%, the African's production increased in 67.73%, the European's production increased in 65.82%, and the American's production with 47.67%. Currently, the world production is dominated by the USA, China, Brazil, Mexico, Russia, and India [4, 14]. The growing demand of meat is proportional to the increasing number of inhabitants in the world and their rising acquiring power, moreover, to the fact that chicken meat cost is cheaper than other kinds of meat [15].

The poultry industry is still confronted with many diseases like coccidiosis, an intestinal parasitic disease that is considered as one of the most aggressive diseases in poultry, causes strong economic losses, and causes damage in animal health and productivity. The global economic loss has been estimated up to 3 billion dollars worldwide including production losses, prevention, and treatment costs [4, 13, 16, 17]. Losses are mainly due to morbidity as coccidiosis results in reduction in weight gain and egg production additionally to affect the quality of meat by diminishing feed conversion, malabsorption, and maldigestion and further leads to mortality [18]. The poultry industry operation requires that large groups of chickens are kept on the floor at high humidity in warm conditions, appropriate for the development and transmission of the avian coccidia; therefore, the development of novel and natural compounds that control this disease is imperative [19].

3. Etiologic agents of coccidiosis

In poultry, the principal etiologic agents of coccidiosis are obligatory intracellular protozoan parasites of the genus *Eimeria*, subclass Coccidia that belong to family Eimeriidae and the phylum Apicomplexa [2, 18, 20]. This phylum groups many other protozoa of medical and/or veterinary importance. It has been reported around 5000 species of apicomplexan parasites, including some that affect humans as malarial parasites *Plasmodium* spp.; the zoonotic organisms *Cryptosporidium parvum* and *Toxoplasma gondii*; *Babesia* and *Theileria* and the more recently described *Neospora caninum*, cattle parasites; and *Eimeria* spp., with host diversity as cattle and poultry pathogens [4, 18, 21]. The majority of apicomplexans are obligate intracellular parasites that infect new host cells by invasive extracellular stages, that involve a specialized array of cytoskeletal elements and secretory organelles known as the apical complex (micronemes, rhoptries, dense granules, and conoid and polar rings), and that would provide the structural stability necessary during the host invasion process [4, 18, 21, 22].

On the other hand, a single host species was reported for more 1200 *Eimeria* spp., and all of these are restricted to this single species [3, 23]. Also, close to ten *Eimeria* spp. have been reported that can infect *Gallus gallus var. domesticus*: *E. mitis* [26], *E. maxima* [26], *E. brunetti* [27], *E. acervulina* [24–26], *E. mivati* [28], *E. necatrix* [29], *E. praecox* [29], *E. tenella* [30], and *E. hagani* [31]. In chicken production, seven *Eimeria* spp. that are associated with clinical coccidiosis have been reported: *E. maxima, E. brunetti, E. acervulina, E. tenella, E. praecox, E. necatrix,* and *E. mitis.* Of all these, *E. tenella* causes significant economic losses; therefore, it is the most studied strain [32, 33].

4. Pathogenicity

Eimeria spp. can infect and duplicate inside the mucosal epithelia in several areas of bird by oral means. Subsequently, they cause gut harm (e.g., hemorrhage, diarrhea, inflammation, etc.), morbidity, and mortality in poultry [4, 5]. Each of which species of parasite causes disease. But the clinical signs vary according to the species, and their pathogenicity varies in birds of different genetic backgrounds in a range from mild damage to severe damage, i.e., are considered highly pathogenic: *E. tenella, E. maxima, E. necatrix,* and *E. brunetti* that has been well characterized in relationship of the neurotic conditions they create, furthermore, the gross lesions that are found in several areas of the gut, however, *E. mitis* and *E. acervulina* do not produce gross lesions or cause mortality in infected host, for their tissue trophism, therefore, are considered mildly pathogenic, whereas *E. praecox* is considered to be the least pathogenic, although in *Eimeria* high densities population levels can potentially cause illness (**Table 1**) [5, 33–35].

Eimeria species	Site of development	Oocyst size (μm)		Shape	Gross lesions	Pathogenicity	Ref.
		Length	Width				
E. necatrix	Jejunum, ileum, ceca	12–29	11–24	Ovoid	The intestine may be ballooned The mucosa thickened and the lumen filled with fluid, blood, and tissue debris Lesions in dead birds are observable as black and white plaques (schizont accumulations)	++++	[4, 29, 43, 44]
E. tenella	Ceca	14–31	9–25	Ovoid	Thickened cecal wall and bloody contents at the proximal end Distension of cecum Villi of the duodenum destruction causing extensive hemorrhage and death	++++	[4, 30, 43–45]
E. brunetti	Ceca, rectum	14–34	12–26	Ovoid	Inflammation of the intestinal wall with pinpointed hemorrhages Sloughing of epithelia	++++	[4, 27, 43, 44]
E. maxima	Jejunum, ileum,	21–42	16–30	Ovoid	Inflammation of the intestinal wall with pinpointed hemorrhages Sloughing of epithelia	+++	[4, 26, 43, 44]
E. mitis	Ileum	10–21	9–18	Subspherical	Limited enteritis causing fluid loss Malabsorption of nutrients	++	[4, 26, 43, 44]
E. acervulina	Duodenum, ileum	12–23	9–17	Ovoid	Limited enteritis causing fluid loss Malabsorption of nutrients Small red spots and white bands on the upper part of the small intestine	++	[4, 26, 43, 44]
E. praecox	Jejunum, duodenum	20–25	16–20	Ovoid	Watery intestinal contents Mucus and mucoid casts	+	[4, 29, 43, 46]

Table 1. Important characteristics of ***Eimeria*** ssp. which are causative agent of coccidiosis.

5. Clinical signs and lesions

Birds infected with coccidiosis show signs like huddling, listlessness, diarrhea, loss of appetite, and weight loss [36]. Many *Eimeria* spp. are able to cause observable clinical signs to infected and unprotected birds; nevertheless, however, it is frequently determined by subclinical infections. These are often undervalued but frequently result in impaired feed conversion and reduced weight gain [37].

Young birds are more susceptible and easily display signs of disease; in contrast, older chickens are relatively resistant as a result of prior infection. The factors that influencing on the severiry of infections are the number of *Eimeria* spp. sporulated oocysts ingested, age of birds, and immune and environmental status of the group; in addition, the contagion can be aggravated because the infected birds tend to huddle together, and droppings are whitish or bloody and watery, ending with dehydration and poor weight gain as well as mortalities [37].

Many different *Eimeria* spp. can infect several areas of the intestinal mucosa and infringe a degree of epithelial cell damage like inflammation [38]. The damage of coccidiosis infection is measured by the degree of inflammation and damage to the intestinal tract: petechial hemorrhages, necrosis, mucous profuse bleeding in the ceca, and mucoid to blood-tinged exudates (**Table 1**).

The tissue harm in the intestinal tract may permit other colonizations by different microorganisms, for example, *Clostridium perfringens* [39]. It has been reported that the infection for *Histomonas meleagridis* was more severe when combined with *E. tenella* [37, 40]. The damage leads to dehydration, diarrhea, dysentery, rectal prolapse, and death [41]. Moreover, each *Eimeria* sp. varies in infection location in the gastrointestinal tract (ranging from the duodenum to the cecum). For example, *E. mitis* infects in the middle part of the small intestine, *E. necatrix* infects in the small intestine, *E. acervulina* infects in the duodenum, *E. maxima* and *E. tenella* infect in the ceca, and *E. brunetti* develops in the ceca and the rectum (**Table 1**) [5, 33, 42].

6. Life cycle

The biological cycle of the protozoa of the genus *Eimeria* is similar to that of other protozoans of the coccidial type. They are obligate intracellular parasites that infect and develop in epithelial cells of the intestinal mucosa causing severe damage to the gut [47]. The life cycles of *Eimeria* spp. are complex, include three different phases, sporogony, merogony, and gametogony, and comprise both sexual and asexual reproductive phases [35, 48]. Some species vary in the number of asexual generations and in the time corresponding to every developmental stage [13, 49].

Infections begin when sporozoites are released from sporocyst and penetrate new cells. Once the sporozoite has achieved to penetrate into the epithelial cell, it forms the vacuola parasitofora and undergoes a process of rounding, transforming into a trophozoite. Then, by multiple nuclear divisions (so-called schizogony), the trophozoites become in the schizonts of the first generation. At the end of the maturation of the schizont, rupture of the membrane of the cell host allows the release of the merozoites to penetrate new cells [50].

These cycles of asexual schizogony (merogony) may be repeated numerous times. The sporozoites undergo merogony resulting in the release from one sporozoite of about 1,000 merozoites; occasionally, this stage is repeated two to four times and after sometimes merozoites develop into either male or female and form into host cell (gametogony, the sexual phase) [33, 50]. Microgametes (male) are flagellated and travel to the immobile macrogametes (female) to fertilize these stages. Upon fertilization, the wall-forming bodies of the macrogametes are externalized and fuse to form the oocyst wall of the unsporulated oocyst that is released from the intestinal mucosa and then is excreted with the feces [4, 33, 49–53].

Once the birds are infected, sporozoites are released within oocysts and penetrate new host cells in the intestinal mucosa, to invade and destroy them and initiate the life cell cycle. As a consequence, infected birds display symptoms of disease such as reduced feed intake, bloody diarrhea, hampered weight gain, loss of appetite, and huddling [2, 4, 36, 50, 54]. The complete process between oocyst ingestion and release may take between 4 and 6 days (depending on the species) [49].

Pathogenic species are typically characterized by at least one large endogenous life cycle stage, which may be asexual (e.g., second-generation schizont of *E. tenella* or *E. necatrix*) or gametocyte (e.g., *E. maxima*). The prepatent period usually fluctuates from 4 to 5 days after oral infection, and maximal oocyst output ranges from day 6 to 9 post-infection [52].

7. Modes of transmission

Coccidian parasites are transmitted by direct or indirect contact with the excrement of other infected birds; afterward a bird ingests coccidia, the organism invades the intestinal mucosa causing damages in the tissues as it reproduces [50, 55]. Following infection, coccidia produces immature oocytes, which are expelled with the fecal matter, usually in an unsporulated (no infective state) and cannot infect another bird unless they undergo a process of sporulation (infective state). Oocysts may remain in the environment for months to years, depending on the species and environmental conditions [50]. In the environment, sporozoites are protected from desiccation, as well as climatic conditions, such as cold, hot weather, and chemical disinfection by the oocyst wall. This structure assures successful disease transmission and is essential for the parasite survival in the environment [50, 55]. In this regard, it has been reported that in environmental conditions the sporulated oocyst can survive up to 602 days, while an unsporulated oocyst can survive up to 7 months in the cecal tissue [4, 33].

8. Coccidian oocysts

A defining characteristic of the *Coccidia* spp. is the development of resistant oocysts that are shed with feces. The coccidian oocyst are exogenous stages that are usually unsporulated in the feces and are considered a remarkably hard and persistent structure. It is resistant to mechanical and chemical damage and to proteolytic degradation. They are difficult to eliminate from the environment because they are surrounded by an indestructible wall that confers resistance to chemical disinfection [55–57].

Plant	Compound	Species	Life cycle stages	Reference
Artemisia annua	Artemisinin	*E. tenella*	Oocyst formation	[58, 59]
		E. acervulina	Sporulated	
		E. máxima		
Pinus radiata	Tannin	*E. tenella*	Sporulated	[60]
		E. acervulina		
		E. máxima		
Azadirachta indica	Bornyl acetate	*E. tenella*	Oocyst formation (immune modulation)	[61, 62]
	α-Pinene limonene			
	b-Caryophyllene			
Sophora flavescens	2-Ethyl-1-hexanol geranyl	*E. tenella*	Oocyst formation (immune modulation)	[63, 64]
		E. acervulina		
		E. máxima		
Berberis lycium	Berberine	*E. tenella*	Oocyst formation (immune modulation)	[65–67]
	Berberine palmitine	*E. acervulina*		
	Antocyanin berbamine	*E. maxima*		
Origanum vulgare	Thymol	*E. tenella*	Oocyst formation	[68, 69]
	Carvacrol	*E. acervulina*		
	γ-Terpinene	*E. maxima*		
	p-Cymene			
Pimpinella anisum	p-Allylanisole	*E. tenella*	Sporulated	[58]
	Z-a-biosabolene			
Allium sativum	Allicin	*E. tenella*	Sporulated	[70]
Bidens pilosa	Polyacetylene	*E. tenella*	Oocyst formation (immune modulation)	[71]
Linum usitatissimum	N-3fatty acids	*E. tenella*	Schizogony	[72]
Ageratum conyzoides	Flavonoids	*E. tenella*	Schizogony	[73]
Carica papaya	Papain	*E. tenella*	Oocyst formation (immune modulation)	[74]
Syzygium aromaticum	Eugenol and eugenyl acetate	*E. tenella*	Sporulated	[75]
Melaleuca alternifolia	Terpinen-4-ol and gamma-terpinene	*E. oocyst*	Oocyst formation	[75]

Table 2. Anticoccidial activity of plants against *Eimeria* spp. and their target life cycle stage.

Commercial product	Composition	Supplier
Solucox	Vinegar of cider, macerates of red rose (*Rosa gallica*), white thyme (*Thymus vulgare*), goldenrod (*Solidago virga aurea*), oregano (*Origanum vulgare*)	La Ferme de Beaumont
Elan Biotic®	Mixture of plant extracts, herbs, essential oils, organic acids, and tannins	Olus plus BV
Elan plus®	Mixture of plant extracts, herbs, essential oils, organic acids, and tannins	Olus plus BV
Necotyl®	Mixture of plant extracts, herbs, essential oils, organic acids, and tannins	Olus plus BV
Verm-X Poultry® Pellets	Wheat meal, wheatfeed meal, limestone flour, garlic, cinnamon, common thyme, seaweed meal, sunflower oil, nettle, cleavers, fennel, peppermint, slippery elm, quassia, dicalcium phosphate, cayenne	Verm-X
Verm-X Poultry® Liquid	Cinnamon, garlic, common thyme, peppermint, fennel, cleavers, nettle, slippery elm, quassia, elecampane	Verm-X
Cocci-Guard	Concentrated saponin extract	DPI Global
BP formulation	*Bidens pilosa*, and other plants	Ta Fong, Inc.
Alquernat Zycox	Mixture of plants *Holarrhena antidysenterica*, *Berberis aristata*, *Embelia ribes*, and *Acorus calamus*, polyphenols, essential oils, and polysaccharides	Biovet SA
Plant and extracts having anticoccidial activity	Mixture of *Quercus infectoria*, *Rhus chinensis*, and *Terminalia chebula*	Kemin Industries
Apacox	*Agrimonia eupatoria*, *Echinacea angustifolia*, *Embelia ribes*, *nigrum*, *Cinchona succirubra*	GreenVet
Avihicox	*Bocconia cordata* and clove extract	Centaur
Nutrimin	Apple cider vinegar	Chicken Licken
Kocci Free	Free olive leaf, mustard seed, black seed, cloves, grapefruit seed extract	Amber Technology
Oil of oregano factors	Oregano extra virgin olive oil (80% carvacrol)	Natural factors
Oilis	Natural vegetal extracts	Engormix
Oreganico	Oregano oil and essential oils	Flyte so fancy
Garlic	Garlic granules	Flyte So Fancy
Poultry ProVita	Probiotics and prebiotic inulin	Vets Plus
CitriStim®	CitriStim Mannan oligosaccharides and beta glucans	ADM
Orego-Stim®	Orego-Stim carvacrol (82%) and thymol (2.4%)	Saife VetMed
Herban	Etheric oils, soya oils, oregano oils	Uncle Ted's Organics Ltd.
Herb 'n' Thrive	Concentrated blend of herbs and essential oils	Chicken Licken
Eimericox®	Several essential oils (Phytosynthese/Trouw Nutrition)	Phytosynthese/Trouw Nutrition

Commercial product	Composition	Supplier
Natustat	Several essential oils and yeast cell walls	Alltech
EnteroGuard	Garlic and cinnamon	Orffa
Xtract Immunocox	Spanish pepper and turmeric	Pancosma
Coxynil	*Allium sativum* Linn 15%, *Cinnamomum camphora* Nees and Eberum 15%, *Elephantopus scaber* Linn 15%, *Valeriana wallichii* DC 15%, sulfur dioxide 25% and NaCl 15%	Growell India
Ropadiar® (powder and liquid)	Ethereal oil (oregano oil)	Ropapharm
Modified from [4].		

Table 3. Natural products available to control coccidiosis.

9. Prevention and control of coccidiosis

Avian coccidiosis is hard to eradicate by two principal reason: first, the oocyst wall is environmentally resistant and second, the sporulated oocyst can outlive for long time in the environment. Currently, controls strategies mainly depend on the use of anticoccidial drugs and live vaccines but the use of natural compounds to prevent avian coccidiosis go up daily [33].

These natural products can include plant extracts, probiotics. In poultry, mainly used as diet supplements with diverse effects as stimulation of immune response, anti inflammatory activities, cytoplasmic damage and antioxidant. By other hand, natural compounds from plant extracts possess metabolites with distinct mode of action capable to inhibiting different stages of the *Eimeria* species life cycle (**Tables 2** and **3**) [4, 7].

10. Conclusions

Coccidiosis is a frequent cause of diarrhea, morbidity, and mortality in domesticated birds, and notwithstanding a broad number of drugs to control this disease are commercially available. *Eimeria* species have developed resistance to conventional anticoccidial drugs over time. Due to widespread development of resistance and the increase of concern of consumers on food safety, different efforts have been made to search for new agents with anticoccidial activity. In this regard, the investigation on natural alternatives has grown quickly and has been considered the most effective and safe strategy for the control and prevention of coccidiosis. On the other hand, these new strategies are friendly with the environment, so that although they have a higher cost, the advantages that these offer are worth. Finally, recent advances in "omics" provide a novel approach for gene discovery involved in anticoccidial drug resistance and for developing marker-assisted selection strategies like method of disease prevention and control.

Author details

Mayra E. Cobaxin-Cárdenas

Address all correspondence to: cobaxin.mayra@inifap.gob.mx

Anaplasmosis Unit, National Center for Disciplinary Research in Veterinary Parasitology, CENID-PAVET, INIFAP, Jiutepec, Morelos, México

References

[1] De Gussem M. Coccidiosis in poultry: Review on diagnosis, control, prevention and interaction with overall gut health. In: Proceedings of the 16th European Symposium on Poultry Nutrition. 2007. pp. 253-261

[2] Gilbert ER, Cox PM, Williams CM, et al. *Eimeria* species and genetic background influence the serum protein profile of broilers with coccidiosis. PLoS ONE. 2011;**6**(1). Article ID: e14636

[3] Chapman HD, Barta JR, Blake D, Gruber A, Jenkins M, Smith NC, Suo X, Tomley FM.A selective review of advances in coccidiosis research. Advances in Parasitology. 2013;**83**: 93-171

[4] Quiroz-Castañeda RE, Dantán-González E. Control of avian coccidiosis: Future and present natural alternatives. BioMed Research International. 2015;**2015**:11. Article ID: 430610. http://dx.doi.org/10.1155/2015/430610

[5] Shivaramaiah C, Barta JR, Hernandez-Velasco X, Téllez G, Hargis B. Coccidiosis: Recent advancements in the immunobiology of *Eimeria* species, preventive measures, and the importance of vaccination as a control tool against these Apicomplexan parasites. Veterinary Medicine: Research and Reports. 2014;**5**:23-34. DOI: 10.2147/VMRR.S57839

[6] Muthamilselvan T, Kuo TF, Wu YC, Yang WC. Herbal remedies for coccidiosis control: A review of plants, compounds, and anticoccidial actions. Evidence-Based Complementary and Alternative Medicine. 2016;**2016**:19. Article ID: 2657981. http://dx.doi.org/10.1155/2016/2657981

[7] Abbas RZ, Colwell DD, Gilleard J. Botanicals: An alternative approach for the control of avian coccidiosis. World's Poultry Science Journal. 2012;**68**:203-215. DOI: 10.1017/S0043933912000268

[8] Peek HW, Landman WJM. Coccidiosis in poultry: Anticoccidial products, vaccines and other prevention strategies. Veterinary Quarterly. 2011;**31**:143-161. DOI: 10.1080/01652176.2011.605247

[9] Guo FC, Kwakkel RP, Williams BA, Suo X, Li WK, Verstegen MW. Coccidiosis immunization: Effects of mushroom and herb polysaccharides on immune responses of chickens with *Eimeria tenella*. Avian Disease. 2005;**49**:70-73

[10] Guven E, Avcioglu H, Aslan A, Hayirli A. Anticoccidal Efficacy of Usnic Acid in Broilers. Kafkas Üniversitesi Veteriner Fakültesi Dergis. 2016;**22**(4):551-556

[11] Smil V. Worldwide transformation of diets, burdens of meat production and opportunities for novel food proteins. Enzyme and Microbial Technology. 2002;**30**(3):305-311

[12] Bogosavljevic-Boskovic S, Mitrovic S, Djokovic R, Doskovic V, Djermanovic V. Chemical composition of chicken meat produced in extensive indoor and free range rearing systems. African Journal of Biotechnology. 2010;**9**(53):9069-9075

[13] Blake DP, Tomley FM. Securing poultry production from the ever-present *Eimeria* challenge. Trends in Parasitology. 2014;**30**:12-19. DOI: 10.1016/j.pt.2013.10.003

[14] FAOSTAT. 2014. Livestock poultry production. http://faostat.fao.org/

[15] Belova AV, Smutka L, Rosochatecká E. World chicken meta market—Its development and current status. Acta Universitatis Agriculturae et Silviculturae Mendelianae Brunensis. 2012;**60**(4):15-30

[16] Blake DP, Clark EL, Macdonald SE, Thenmozhi V, Kundu K, Garg R, Reid AJ. Population, genetic, and antigenic diversity of the apicomplexan *Eimeria tenella* and their relevance to vaccine development. Proceedings of the National Academy of Science. 2015;**112**(38): E5343-E5350

[17] Dalloul RA, Lillehoj HS. Poultry coccidiosis: Recent advancements in control measures and vaccine development. Expert Review of Vaccines. 2006;**5**(1):143-163

[18] Oz HS. Selective induced altered coccidians to immunize and prevent enteritis. Gastroenterology Research and Practice. 2016;**2016**:8. Article ID: 3952534. http://dx.doi.org/10.1155/2016/3952534

[19] Shirley MW, Smith AL, Tomley FM. The biology of avian *Eimeria* with an emphasis on their control by vaccination. Advances in Parasitology. 2005;**60**:285-330

[20] Ahmad TA, El-Sayed BA, El-Sayed LH. Development of immunization trials against *Eimeria* spp. Trials in Vaccinology. 2016;**5**:38-47

[21] Morrison DA. Evolution of the Apicomplexa: Where are we now? Trends in Parasitology. 2009;**25**(8):375-382

[22] Hu K, Johnson J, Florens L, et al. Cytoskeletal components of an invasion machine the apical complex of *Toxoplasma gondii*. PLoS Pathogens. 2006;**2**(2):e13

[23] Reid AJ, Blake DP, Ansari HR, Billington K, Browne HP, Bryant J, Malas TB. Genomic analysis of the causative agents of coccidiosis in domestic chickens. Genome Research. 2014;**24**(10):1676-1685

[24] Morgan JAT, Morris GM, Wlodek BM, et al. Real time polymerase chain reaction (PCR) assays for the specific detection and quantification of seven *Eimeria* species that cause coccidiosis in chickens. Molecular and Cellular Probes. 2009;**23**(2):83-89

[25] Haug A, Gjevre AG, Thebo P, Mattsson JG, Kaldhusdal M. Coccidial infections in commercial broilers: Epidemiological aspects and comparison of *Eimeria* species identification by morphometric and polymerase chain reaction techniques. Avian Pathology. 2008;**37**(2):161-170

[26] Tyzzer EE. Coccidiosis in gallinaceous birds. American Journal of Hygiene. 1929;**10**: 269-383

[27] Levine PP. A new coccidium pathogenic for chickens, *Eimeria* brunetti n. sp. (Protozoa: Eimeriidae). Cornell. Veterinarian. 1942;**32**:430-439

[28] Edgar SA, Siebold CT. A New coccidium of chickens, *Eimeria* mivati sp. n. (Protozoa: Eimeriidae), with details of its life history. Journal of Parasitology. 1964;**50**:193-204

[29] Johnson WT. Coccidiosis of the chicken with special reference to species. Standard Bulletin Oregon Agriculture Experiment station. 1938;**358**:3-33

[30] Raillet A, Lucet A. Note sur quelques especes de coccidies encore peu etudiees. Bulletin de la Société Zoologique de France. 1891;**16**:246-250

[31] Levine PP. *Eimeria* hagani n. sp. (Protozoa: Eimeriidae) a new coccidium of the chicken. Cornell Veterinarian. 1938;**28**:263-266

[32] Williams RB. A compartmentalised model for the estimation of the cost of coccidiosis to the world's chicken production industry. International Journal for Parasitology. 1999;**29**:1209-1229

[33] Price KR. Use of live vaccines for coccidiosis control in replacement layer pullets. Journal of Applied Poultry Research. 2012;**21**(3):679-692

[34] Jadhav BN, Nikam SV, Bhamre SN, Jaid EL. Study of *Eimeria* necatrix in broiler chicken from Aurangabad district of Maharashtra state India. International Multidisciplinary Research Journal. 2011;**1**(11):11-12

[35] Lillehoj HS. Influence of inoculation dose, inoculation schedule, chicken age, and host genetics on disease susceptibility and development of resistance to *Eimeria tenella* infection. Avian Diseases. 1988;**32**:437-444

[36] McDonald V, Shirley MW. Past and future: Vaccination against *Eimeria*. Parasitology. 2009;**136**(12):1477-1489

[37] Hafez HM. Poultry coccidiosis: Prevention and control approaches. Archiv fur Geflugelkunde. 2008;**72**(1):2-7

[38] Finlay RC, Roberts SJ, Hayday AC. Dynamic response of murine gut intraepithelial T cells after infection by the coccidian parasite *Eimeria*. European Journal of Immunology. 1993;**23**:2557-2564

[39] Helmbolt CF, Bryant ES. The pathology of necrotic enteritis in domestic fowl. Avian Diseases. 1971;**15**:775-780

[40] McDougald LR, Hu J. Blackhead disease (*Histomonas meleagridis*) aggravated in broiler chickens by concurrent infection with cecal coccidiosis (*Eimeria tenella*). Avian Diseases. 2001;**45**:307-312

[41] Cook GC. Small intestinal coccidiosis: And emergent clinical problem. Journal of Infection. 1988;**16**:213-219

[42] Raman M, Banu SS, Gomathinayagam S, Raj GD. Lesion scoring technique for assessing the virulence and pathogenicity of Indian field isolates of avian *Eimeria* species. Veterinarski Archive. 2011;**81**(2):259-271

[43] Peek HW, Landman WJM. Coccidiosis in poultry: Anticoccidial products and alternative prevention strategies (a review). Veterinary Quarterly, 31;**3**:143-161. http://dx.doi.org/10.1080/01652176.2011.605247

[44] Chapman HD. Milestones in avian coccidiosis research: A review. Poultry Science. 2014;**93**(3):501-511

[45] Duffy CF, Mathis GF, Power RF. Effects of Natustat supplementation on performance, feed efficiency and intestinal lesion scores in broiler chickens challenged with *Eimeria acervulina, Eimeria maxima* and *Eimeria tenella*. Veterinary Parasitology. 2005;**130**(3-4):185-190

[46] McDougald LR, Fitz-Coy SH. Protozoal infections. In: Saif YM, editor. Diseases of Poultry. Ames, Iowa, USA: Blackwell Publishing; 2009. p. 1352

[47] Min W, Dalloul RA, Lillehoj HS. Application of biotechnological tools for coccidia vaccine development. Journal of Veterinary Science. 2004;**5**(4):279-288

[48] Hammond DM. Life cycles and development of coccidian. In: Hammond DM, Long PL, editors. The Coccidia. Baltimore, MD: University Park Press; 1982. pp. 45-79

[49] McDougald LR. Coccidiosis. In: Swayne DE, editor. Diseases of Poultry. Wiley-Blackwell; 2013. p. 1408

[50] Barta JR. Coccidiosis. Encyclopedia of Life Sciences. 2001;**19**(April):1-8. DOI: 10.1038/npg.els.0001947

[51] Seemann E, Kurth T, Entzeroth R. Insight into the ultrastructural organisation of sporulated oocysts of *Eimeria* nieschulzi (Coccidia, Apicomplexa). Parasitology Research. 2012;**111**:2143-2147

[52] Reid WM, Long PL. A diagnostic chart for nine species of fowl coccidia. In: Bowen NB, editor. Georgia Agric. Exp. Stn. Tech. Bull. Athens: College of Agriculture, University of Georgia; 1979. pp. 5-24

[53] Kheysin YM. Sporulation of oocysts and their survival in the external environment. In: Todd Jr KS, editor. Life Cycles of Coccidia of Domestic Animals. Baltimore, MD: University Park Press; 1972;**33**:149-161

[54] Dalloul RA, Lillehoj HS. Recent advances in immunomodulation and vaccination strategies against coccidiosis. Avian Diseases. 2005;**49**(1):1-8

[55] Belli SI, Smith NC, Ferguson DJ. The coccidian oocyst: A tough nut to crack! Trends in Parasitology. 2006;**22**(9):416-423

[56] Kreier JP, editor. Parasitic Protozoa. Vol. 10. San Diego (California): Academic Press. 2013. pp. 225-422

[57] Mai K, Sharman PA, Walker RA, Katrib M, Souza DD, McConville MJ, Smith NC. Oocyst wall formation and composition in coccidian parasites. Memorias do Instituto Oswaldo Cruz. 2009;**104**(2):281-289

[58] Drăgan L, Titilincu A, Dan I, Dunca I, Drăgan M, Mircean V. Effects of *Artemisia annua* and *Pimpinella anisum* on *Eimeria tenella* (Phylum Apicomplexa) low infection in chickens. Scientia Parasitologica. 2010;**11**(2):77-82

[59] del Cacho E, Gallego M, Francesch M, Quílez J, Sánchez-Acedo C. Effect of artemisinin on oocyst wall formation and sporulation during *Eimeria tenella* infection. Parasitology International. 2010;**59**(4):506-511

[60] Molan AL, Liu Z, De S. Effect of pine bark (Pinus radiata) extracts on sporulation of coccidian oocysts. Folia Parasitologica. 2009;**56**(1):1

[61] Biu AA, Yusuf SD, Rabo JS. Use of neem (*Azadirachta indica*) aqueous extract as a treatment for poultry coccidiosis in Borno State Nigeria. African Scientist. 2006;**7**:147-153

[62] Pandey IP, Ahmed SF, Chhimwal S, Pandey S. Chemical composition and wound healing activity of volatile oil of leaves of *Azadirachta indica* A. juss. Advances in Pure and Applied Chemistry. 2012;**1**:62-66

[63] Sundar SB, Harikrishnan TJ, Latha BR, Sarath G, Kumar CTS. Anticoccidial drug resistance in chicken coccidiosis and promising solutions: A review. Journal of Entomology and Zoology Studies. 2017;**5**(4):1526-1529

[64] Li A, Han L, Han CC. Antioxidant and neuroprotective activities of essential oil, isolated from *Chinese herb* pairs of *angelica sinensis* and *sophora flavescens*. Journal of Applied Pharmaceutical Science. 2012;**2**(5):01-04. DOI: 10.7324/JAPS.2012.2505

[65] Malik TA, Kamili AN, Chishti MZ, Tanveer S, Ahad S, Johri RK. *In vivo* anticoccidial activity of berberine [18, 5, 6-dihydro-9, 10-dimethoxybenzo (g)-1, 3-benzodioxolo (5, 6-a) quinolizinium]–an isoquinoline alkaloid present in the root bark of *Berberis lycium*. Phytomedicine. 2014;**21**(5):663-669

[66] Nidaullah H, Durrani FR, Ahmad S, Jan IU, Gul S. Aqueous extract from different medicinal plants as anticoccidial, growth promotive and immunostimulant in broilers. Journal of Agricultural and Biological Science. 2010;**5**(1):53-59

[67] Shabbir A, Shahzad M, Arfat Y, Ali L, Aziz RS, Murtaza G, Waqar SA. Berberis lycium Royle: A review of its traditional uses, phytochemistry and pharmacology. African Journal of Pharmacy and Pharmacology. 2012;**6**(31):2346-2353

[68] Waldenstedt L. Effect of vaccination against coccidiosis in combination with an antibacterial oregano (*Origanum vulgare*) compound in organic broiler production. Acta Agriculturae Scandinavica, Section A-Animal Science. 2003;**53**(2):101-109

[69] D'Antuono LF, Galletti GC, Bocchini P. Variability of essential oil content and composition of *Origanum vulgare* L. populations from a North Mediterranean Area (Liguria Region, Northern Italy). Annals of Botany. 2000;**86**(3):471-478

[70] Alnassan AA, Thabet A, Daugschies A, Bangoura B. *In vitro* efficacy of allicin on chicken *Eimeria tenella* sporozoites. Parasitology Research. 2015;**114**(10):3913-3915

[71] Yang WC, Tien YJ, Chung CY, Chen YC, Chiou WH, Hsu SY, et al. Effect of *Bidens pilosa* on infection and drug resistance of *Eimeria* in chickens. Research in Veterinary Science. 2015;**98**:74-81

[72] Allen PC, Danforth HARRY, Levander OA. Interaction of dietary flaxseed with coccidia infections in chickens. Poultry Science. 1997;**76**(6):822-827

[73] Nweze NE, Obiwulu IS. Anticoccidial effects of Ageratum conyzoides. Journal of Ethnopharmacology. 2009;**122**(1):6-9

[74] Al-Fifi ZIA. Effect of leaves extract of *Carica papaya, Vernonia amigdalina* and *Azadiratcha indica* on the coccidiosis in free-range chickens. Asian Journal of Animal Sciences. 2007;**1**(1):26-32

[75] Remmal A, Achahbar S, Bouddine L, Chami N, Chami F. *In vitro* destruction of *Eimeria* oocysts by essential oils. Veterinary Parasitology. 2011;**182**(2):121-126

Chapter 9

Zoonotic Trematodiasis

Estefan Miranda Miranda

Additional information is available at the end of the chapter

http://dx.doi.org/10.5772/intechopen.72632

Abstract

Parasitic zoonoses are diseases caused by parasites shared between animal hosts and humans. Most of parasitic zoonoses are considered as neglected because of the absence of campaigns destined to prevention control and treatment of these diseases in most developed and undeveloped nations, ignoring that parasitic zoonoses affect almost half of the world human population and the vast majority of livestock worldwide is at risk of acquiring or sick because of a zoonotic disease. Zoonotic trematodiasis are numerous in almost every nation and responsible for serious and debilitating helminthic diseases in about 75 million people as well as the billions of dollars in production losses to the livestock industry. The perspective of global warming, habitat loss and new host range adaptation indicates that unless a new approach based in genomics, transcriptomics and proteomics assessment of new biomarkers and anthelmintic targets is achieved, the incidence of zoonotic trematodiasis will increase for both human and animal hosts.

Keywords: zoonoses, emerging diseases, trematodes, parasites, disease, diagnostics

1. Introduction

Parasitic zoonoses affect almost half of the world's population and cause billions of dollars in losses to the livestock industry. Under the current trend of climate change, wild habitat loss, intensive agriculture-aquiculture activities combined with human demographic increase, zoonotic parasites represent a constant health threat for people and livestock living in most of the developing nations with a deficient or nonexisting healthcare policies or infrastructure [1].

Among zoonotic infections, most of those caused by parasitic pathogens are considered as neglected by the World Health Organization (WHO), in part because these diseases are endemic in undeveloped nations, which cannot afford to allocate economical resources destined to diagnosis prevention and control of at least the most important zoonoses affecting their inhabitants and livestock [2].

The situation is aggravated by a pharmaceutical industry reluctant to invest in research and development efforts for new pharmaceutical treatments in countries that are not a profitable market place [3], resulting in a lack of efficient treatments for the most important parasitic zoonoses around the globe. Zoonotic diseases are those naturally exchanged between vertebrate animals and humans [4], and several modes of zoonotic diseases were identified according to direction of transmission, number of hosts and types of symptoms, definitions of which are indicated in **Table 1**.

Natural habitat invasion by livestock and people are considered the most important detonator for the emergence of zoonotic outbreaks worldwide (**Figure 1**) [5].

Terminology	Definition
Zoonoses	Diseases naturally transmitted between vertebrate animals and humans
Anthropozoonoses	Diseases in animals that can be transmitted to man
Zooanthroponoses	Diseases affecting humans that can be transmitted to animals
Amphixenoses	Diseases that are exchanged between animals and human occasionally
Euzoonoses	Diseases in which humans are an obligatory host of the pathogen
Cyclozoonoses	Diseases that require two different vertebrate hosts but no invertebrate vector
Pherozoonoses	Pherozoonoses isosymptomatic, similar symptoms are observed in animals and humans
	Pherozoonoses anisosymptomatic, symptoms are different in animals and humans
Cryptozoonoses	Zoonotic diseases in which symptoms are only evident in humans
Saprozoonoses	Diseases that depend upon inanimate reservoirs and vertebrate hosts
Emerging parasitic zoonoses	Zoonotic diseases caused either by new parasites or by old known species in an area where the disease was previously unknown

Table 1. Modes of zoonotic diseases identified according to direction of transmission, number of hosts and types of symptoms.

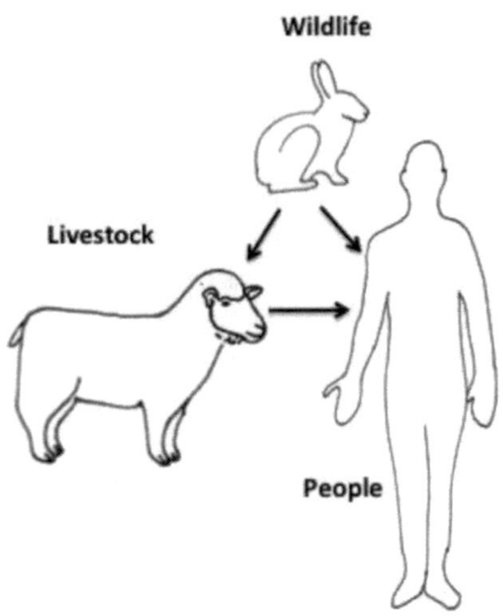

Figure 1. Zoonotic parasite flow among wildlife, livestock, and humans. A condition such as wild habitat invasion by livestock and humans is a major factor in the emergence of a parasitic zoonosis.

http://dx.doi.org/10.5772/intechopen.72632

Some of the most important zoonoses are those caused by well-known pathogens, imported from endemic areas to new ones where the diseases that cause those parasites have not being previously documented. This phenomenon, called "infectious emerging diseases" by the WHO, is defined as newly recognized or newly evolved or that has occurred previously but shows an increase in incidence or expansion in geographical, host, or vector range [6].

Neglected emerging diseases cause around 75% of human infectious diseases worldwide [7, 8]. Parasitic zoonosis, include protozoans and helminths, such as nematodes, cestodes, and trematodes, some of which, exhibit very complex life cycles that require invertebrate vectors that may look as innocuous as a garden snail but instead could be extremely dangerous vectors of very serious and debilitating parasitic diseases. **Table 2** depicts some of the most important parasitic zoonoses, its transmission vehicle and distribution.

Phylum	Genus	Disease	Species	Vector/transmission vehicle	Distribution	Hosts
Protozoa	*Trypanosoma* spp.	American trypanosomiasis	*T. cruzi*	Triatomid bugs	All American countries except Canada	Ruminants Canines Cats Marsupials Humans
		African trypanosomiasis	*T. brucei*	Glossina flies	African countries	Ruminants Canines Cats Humans
	Leishmania spp.	Middle East leishmaniasis	*L. donovani*	Plebotomid flies	Middle and Far East countries	Ruminants Canines Cats Humans
		American leishmaniasis	*L. mexicana* *L. brasiliensis* *L. tropica*	Plebotomid flies	Meso American tropical and subtropical countries	Ruminants Canines Cats Humans
	Cryptosporidium spp.	Cryptosporidiosis	*C. parvum*	Food and waterborne	Worldwide	Aquatic fowl Humans
	Toxoplasma spp.	Toxoplasmosis	*T. gondii*	Cat feces raw meat	Worldwide	Ruminants Canines Cats, birds, reptiles, humans
Nematoda	*Ancylostoma* spp.	Hookworm disease	*A. duodenale*	Skin penetration	Worldwide	Canines Humans
	Ascaris spp.	Roundworm disease	*A. suum*	Foodborne Pig feces	Worldwide	Pigs Humans
	Toxocara spp.	Toxocariasis	*T. canis*	Foodborne Dog feces	Worldwide	Dogs Cats Humans
	Strongyloides spp.	Strongyloidiasis	*S. stercoralis*	Skin penetration	Worldwide	Dogs Humans
	Dirofilaria spp.	Heart Filariasis	*D. immitis*	Mansonia, Anopheles and Aedes mosquitoes	Worldwide	Dogs Humans
	Brugia spp.	Lymphatic filariasis	*B. malayi*	Mansonia, Anopheles and Aedes mosquitoes	Southeast Asia	

Phylum	Genus	Disease	Species	Vector/transmission vehicle	Distribution	Hosts
						Dogs, cats Monkeys and humans
Platyhelminths Cestoda	*Hymenolepis* spp.	Dwarf tapeworm disease	*H. nana*	Foodborne	Worldwide	Rodents Humans
	Dipylidium spp.	Flea tapeworm disease	*D. caninum*	Accidental flea ingestion	Worldwide	Cats Dogs Humans
	Diphyllobothrium spp.	Fish tapeworm disease	*D. latum*	Raw fish	Worldwide	Fish Ichtyophagus mammals Humans
	Taenia spp.	Pig tapeworm disease	*T. solium*	Raw pork	Worldwide	Pigs Humans
		Cow tapeworm disease	*T. saginata*	Raw beef	Worldwide	Bovines Humans
Platyhelminths Trematoda	*Fasciola* spp.	Liver fluke	*F. hepatica* *F. gigantica*	Snail. Fresh vegetables	Worldwide	Ruminants Pigs Rodents Humans
	Fasciolopsis spp.	Giant intestinal fluke	*F. buski*	Snail. Fresh vegetables	Southeast Asia	Pigs Humans
	Clonorchis spp.	Chinese liver fluke	*C. sinensis*	Snail. Fish	Southeast Asia	Pigs Cats Canines Ruminants Humans
	Schistosoma spp.	Cercarial dermatitis	Nonhuman *Schistosoma* spp.	Waterborne	Worldwide	Birds Most mammals Humans
	Paragonimus spp.	Lung fluke	*P. westermani* *P. mexicanus*	Snail, crustaceans	Southeast Asia Central America	Cats Canines Rodents Humans
Arthropoda	*Sarcoptes* spp.	Scabies	*S. scabiei*	Direct contact	Worldwide	Dogs Humans
	Trombicula spp.	Trombiculosis	*T. alfreddugesi*	Direct contact	North America	Mammals Birds Humans
	Ixodes spp.	Deer tick	*I. scapularis*	Direct contact	North America	Mammals Humans

Table 2. Important global parasitic zoonoses.

2. Zoonotic trematodes life cycle and transmission

Zoonotic parasites are transmitted to livestock and people using well-known routes, these may include blood sucking invertebrate vectors such as the sand flies role in transmitting river blindness, foodborne like in the case of zoonotic trematodiasis or direct contact with wildlife

http://dx.doi.org/10.5772/intechopen.72632

and/or domestic animals such as in the case of scabies [9]. Human zoonotic helminthiasis are of particular importance because of their insidious nature, showing a tendency to increase for a number of factors, most notably global population growth and global warming trends [7].

Part of the emergence of zoonotic parasites is due to the climate change expectative [10–12], and climate change may disrupt vertebrate and invertebrate hosts or their habitat, increasing contact with human population and livestock or favoring conditions of vector proliferation [13]. When livestock and aquiculture is considered as additional factors, the risk to human health increases dramatically due to the inability of most undeveloped nations to put in place efficient methods of vertebrate-invertebrate hosts control, resulting in high prevalence of zoonotic helminthiasis among farmers and fisheries workers [14].

Zoonotic trematodiasis depends on several species of gastropod mollusks to complete their life cycle. Part of the successful conquest of new habitats depends on the adaptation of the different parasitic trematodes to new intermediate hosts around the world (**Figure 2**) [15]. This is the case of *Fasciola* spp. parasitic trematodes, which spread from Europe to the rest of the world by adapting to *Radix* sp., *Bithynia* sp., and new species of *Lymnaea* sp. slimes in the American countries [16].

Intermediate host adaptation is an important factor in the emergence of a neglected disease where endemicity is low or nonexistent. Food-borne trematode zoonoses (FBTZ) start their life cycle as miracidium, a 100-micrometer ciliated developmental stage result of trematodes embryonated eggs, highly mobile in aquatic conditions, upon finding a compatible snail, the miracidium penetrates the tegument of the intermediate host shedding its cilia [17] turning into germinal masses of cells called sporocysts.

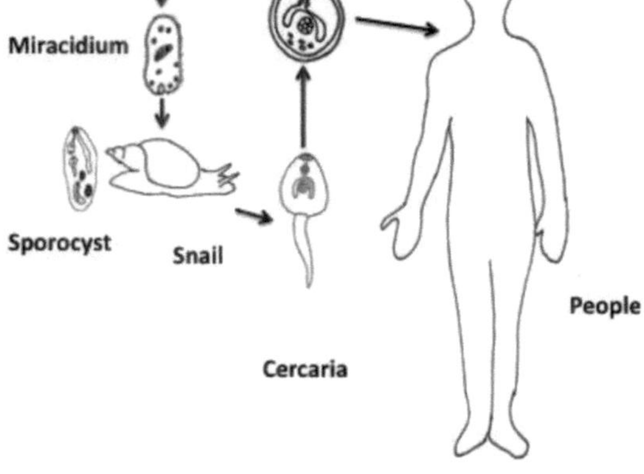

Figure 2. Life cycle of zoonotic trematodes.

These sporocysts multiply into several masses of germinal cell each of them originating a redia [18], and these are intermediate germinal stages that develop into cercariae, a highly mobile developmental stage that finally exits the intermediate host by perforation of the snail's tegument and then migrates into an aquatic environment, the cercariae, depending on the parasitic trematode species, can penetrate the skin of a second intermediate host and encyst in the muscles of it [19]. Cercariae may also penetrate the skin of the definitive host [6] or lose its tail and become a cyst, an environment-resistant developmental stage on surrounding vegetation or in drinking water. Cercariae and metacercariae are the infestant stage of zoonotic trematodes, and upon ingestion or penetration, they grow into a juvenile worm [20]. Alternative infestation modes have being reported [6] in places where row meat consumption is common, accidental ingestion of juvenile/adult flukes can occur, a phenomenon known as paratenic trematodiasis [7].

Once established in their target organs, parasitic trematodes may induce a chronic trematodiasis producing a serious illness that may last decades [21]. Livestock may carry zoonotic trematodiasis during their entire life span within endemic areas, and several definitive hosts have been reported such as American and Asian camelids, rodents, deer, hare, and pigs [22].

3. Socioeconomic impact and distribution

Trematode zoonoses are neglected diseases mostly due to the lack of funds required for diagnosis prevention and control of zoonotic parasites [5]. Trematode zoonosis include the liver, intestinal and lung flukes [20] and are endemic worldwide; although they can be found in developed nations, the most important socioeconomic impact occurs in undeveloped nations where around 750 million people are at risk of acquiring trematodiasis [23], most cases related to clonorchiasis, paragonimiasis, fascioliasis, and opisthorchiasis [23].

SouthEast Asian countries are the most affected with clonorchiasis estimated as 35 million people [24] followed by paragonimiasis and opisthorchiasis with 20 and 10 million affected humans, respectively [25]. *Fasciola* sp. trematodiasis affects some 17 million people globally and a large amount of livestock constituting both a world health problem and livestock production issue [22]. Intestinal flukes mostly due to *Fasciolopsis burki* are estimated to affect some 50 million inhabitants [26]. Human trematodiasis occurs via water or food products contaminated by the intermedian host that may be fish, mollusks, or vegetables [16]. Part of the social and economic importance of FBTZ is the fact that several animal species are also affected, which makes these kinds of diseases a veterinary issue as well as a human health problem [6].

Fasciola hepatica is the causative agent of fascioliasis, a debilitating parasitic disease that destroys the hepatic parenchyma and blocks the bile ducts of equines, bovines, swine, sheep, goats, rabbits, and humans [27]. Fascioliasis is considered a neglected zoonotic parasitic disease, because it is ignored by most countries where fascioliasis is endemic, in spite of 91 million more human beings at risk of acquiring fascioliasis in endemic areas, where 2.4 million new human cases are reported each year [28, 29].

Latin America, human fascioliasis is dangerously neglected by the official health system and as in many other neglected diseases, there is no collection of the most basic epidemiological figures on the subject and only sporadic clinical reports are found on the medical literature

[30]. High rates of ovine and bovine fascioliasis prevalence are reported in Latin American countries slaughterhouses, and the livestock industry worldwide reports annual losses of 4 billion dollars associated with poor conversion of livestock feed into meat, wool and milk, low weight gain, and reduced fertility [29, 31].

The veterinary impact of zoonotic parasitic food-borne trematodiasis is mainly economical due to loss of animal products of the affected livestock [13]. Cercarial dermatitis is an aberrant form of zoonotic trematodiasis caused by several avian parasitic trematodes or *Schistosoma* spp., and it may occur anywhere around the planet and on a seasonal basis with most cases reported during the summer time [32]. It happens when the invertebrate intermediate hosts or snails releases cercariae in water ponds coinciding with human activities such as recreational swimming or fishing [33], aquiculture and agricultural such as rice planting activities are also important occupational risk factors [34]. In these environments, where there are abundance of cercariae, they tend to penetrate any warm blooded vertebrate including people, and thousands of cases are reported each year in North America, Europe, and Asia [33].

4. Emerging zoonotic diseases

Zoonotic trematodiases are also emerging diseases due to the inevitable spread of the intermediate host to new habitats and global warming and increasing activities of aquiculture, representing a threat to new populated areas where zoonotic trematodiasis was not previously documented [15] (**Table 3**).

Most of zoonotic trematodiasis affected areas are located in tropical and subtropical areas where tropical neglected diseases are endemic in coincidence with the world poorest nations where health care is nonexistent and funding for prevention and control of tropical neglected diseases such as parasitic zoonosis is negligible [14]. Respiratory infections, diarrheal diseases, and HIV cases in global health impact only surpass currently zoonotic trematodiasis over the world population [31].

Disease	Intermediate hosts genus	Distribution
Echinostomiasis	*Planorbis* sp. *Lymnaea* sp. *Redix* sp. *Gyraulus* sp. *Hippeutis* sp.	Worldwide
Schistosomiasis	*Bulinus* sp. *Oncomelania* sp. *Biomphalaria* sp. *Neotrícula* sp.	Worldwide
Fascioliasis	*Lymnaea* sp.	Worldwide
Fasciolopsiasis	*Segmentina* sp. *Hippeutis* sp.	
Clororchiasis	*Alocinma* sp. *Bulimus* sp. *Melanoides* sp. *Parafossarulus* sp. Intermedian host: Fish	Worldwide
Dicrocoeliasis	*Cionella* sp. *Bradybaena* sp. snails and *Formica* sp. ants	Worldwide

Table 3. Distribution of invertebrate hosts of different zoonotic trematodes around the world.

Given the high proportion of people at risk of acquiring zoonotic trematodiasis, and the perspective of global warming driving the current situation toward the worst-case scenario, neglected parasitic zoonoses should be addressed as a world health priority by international health organisms [32–35]. Although there have been advances in approaching neglected parasitic zoonoses in recent years, with new treatments and increasing research founding, zoonotic trematodiasis when compared to other zoonoses, remains ignored, in part because of intense competition for the attention and funding of the health organisms and health offices of different developing countries, that are already investing in the control of other high priority neglected diseases [36]. This is also the case for the WHO which has postponed important programs destined to prevention, control and treatment against zoonotic trematodiasis for lack of funding support [37].

Pressure on wild ecosystems adds an important factor for the increase of risk factors of acquiring zoonotic trematodiasis by both animals and human populations. This, mainly due to the destination of new areas for intensive agriculture and livestock production which enable favorable conditions for the proliferation of the intermediate host, and several animal definitive host perpetuating conditions of endemicity in an habitat otherwise unfavorable for parasitic trematodes [37]. Conditions are even worse when aquiculture activities are adopted, increasing transmission hot spots where intermediate host, livestock, and human population converge in a more frequent basis [31]. A description of the zoonotic trematodes invertebrate hosts ubiquity is described in **Table 3**.

5. Anthelmintic resistance

Lung and intestinal trematodiasis are treated with praziquantel, and although some suspicious have emerged regarding the appearance of trematode resistance against this anthelmintic, no solid scientific evidence has been produced so far [35, 38]. On the other hand, fascioliasis is mostly treated with triclabendazole, a halogenated derivative of thiol-benzimidazole [39, 40]. Trematodes metabolize triclabendazole by their xenobiotic metabolizing enzymatic complex (XME). Fascioliasis treatment with triclabendazole has resulted in ever-growing fasciolicide resistance and/or tolerance in several countries around the world [41].

XME complex include enzymes such as Cytochrome P450, alcohol and aldehyde dehydrogenase glutathione S transferases and carboxylesterases [27], which protect trematodes against the toxic action of natural xenobiotics and now are the main defense against synthetic anthelmintic compounds [42]. There is the necessity to use the XME complex as anthelmintic resistance marker and particularly their DNA sequence within their respective genes in order to design fasciolicide resistance diagnostics by DNA technology [28].

Previous comparative transcriptomics in the liver fluke showed that the oxidative metabolic pathway and glutathione-dependent enzymes, which include the XEM complex, exhibited gene overexpression in triclabendazole-resistant *F. hepatica* when cytochrome P450 and glutathione S transferase transcription were assessed [59]. These results suggest that the XME complex is responsible for the transformation of fasciolicides to less toxic bioproducts during the liver fluke's triclabendazole-resistance process [27]. Comparative genomics on *F. hepatica* highlights important changes on the b-tubulin expression, which suggest that the triclabendazole target molecule is playing a role on the liver fluke's anthelmintic resistance [28].

6. Diagnostics and treatment

Most diagnostic procedures of zoonotic trematodiasis start with suspicious symptoms and blood indicators such as eosinophilia [23], and further studies should request for search of eggs in feces, sputum, or urine alone with complementary diagnostics such as hepatobiliary enzyme levels in blood and use of imaging devices like ultrasound or high-resolution nuclear magnetic resonance spectroscopy [43].

The World Health Organization (WHO) has issued several recommendations to countries affected with zoonotic trematodiasis, regarding laboratory procedures of coprology, immunological and molecular diagnostics, as well as treatment prevention and control of zoonotic trematodiasis; WHO also indicates that clinical signs such as hepatomegaly and eosinophilia are clear indicators of trematodiasis [44]. Confirmation, however, relies mostly on the identification of trematodes eggs in feces, urine, or sputum samples [5]. The problem with this diagnostics approach is due to variations of the life cycles of different parasitic trematodes, and most acute clinical signs occur when trematodes are unable to produce eggs, which adds to low sensitivity or reproducibility of the laboratory procedures currently applied [45, 46]. Acute fascioliasis produces liver damage revealed by hepatic enzymes screening in blood and liver imaging; however, juvenile trematodes are not revealed by neither procedure and only 50% of adult flukes are identified [47].

A number of immunological procedures based on hemagglutination, immunofluorescence, and indirect enzyme-linked immunosorbent assay test have been reported as useful both during acute and chronic stages of most trematodiasis [48]. In spite of the success of immunological procedures, most of them rely on the identification of circulating antibodies and are therefore indirect procedures [49]; additionally, blood-circulating antibodies may show high titers long after the elimination of the parasites [53]. For direct confirmation of the causative agent on any zoonotic trematodiasis, some epidemiological studies are carried out by ELISA serological surveys in search for specific blood excretory or secretory antigens [55]. Certain variations of immunodiagnostics search for secretory antigens in fecal samples coupled to an ELISA assay [50], and several other immunological procedures for trematodiasis diagnostics have been developed with mixed results, but in general, trematodiasis may be efficiently diagnosed by immunological procedures with sensitivity of between 89% and 100% [51].

The advancement on the DNA-based technology diagnostic procedures has permitted the applications of PCR diagnostics on feces, urine, and sputum samples in search for trematode specific DNA sequences, PCR depends on parasitic development stages to be present for nucleic acids to be obtained from them, for example: parasitic eggs in fecal or urine samples; a minor disadvantage is that DNA extraction procedures for biological samples, have to be modified in order to obtain a proper amount of nucleic acids for the PCR diagnostics, additionally PCR requires an appropriate set of primers and specialised reagents and equipment which are reviewed

Zoonotic trematodiasis	Parasite	Transmission vehicle	Population at risk (millions)	Estimated cases (millions)	Symptoms	Diagnosis	Treatment
Liver flukes	*Fasciola* spp.	Vegetables	91	17	Fever, diarrhea, loss of appetite, dyspepsia, epigastric pain, nausea, pancreatitis	Eggs detection in feces, Immunodiagnosis. PCR	Triclabendazole
	Clonorchis spp.	Raw fish	601	11			Praziquantel
	Opisthorchis spp.	Raw fish	80	35			
Lung fluke	*Paragonimus* spp.	Crabs, crayfish	292	21	Cough, fever, bloody sputum, chest pain, headache		Praziquantel
Intestinal fluke	*Fasciolopsis buski*	Vegetables	50	Unknown	Diarrhea, constipation, headache, flatulence, loss of appetite, abdominal pain, nausea	Eggs detection in feces, PCR	Praziquantel

Table 4. Zoonotic trematodiasis, public health impact, symptoms, diagnostics, and treatment.

elsewhere [18], however, in spite of these disadvantages, the sensitivity and specificity of this diagnostic test, once performed properly, have no equal when compared to other tests.

7. Genomics of zoonotic trematodiasis

The need for new treatments for zoonotic trematodiasis requires a comprehensive genomics, transcriptomics and proteomics assessment of all parasitic trematodes [60]. Several draft genome efforts are reported for *S. mansoni* [54] and *S. haematobium* [55], similar efforts detailing transcriptomics and proteomics data sets for *S. japonicum* are available [52, 56, 57]. A number of expressed sequence tags have been described for Fish-borne zoonotic trematodes such as *O. viverrini* [58], and the sequence of genes coding for hundreds of important invasive factors are described for *F. hepatica* [28, 59].

As a result of comparative transcriptomics assessment, novel treatments using miRNA interference of invasive factor have shown encouraging results for schistosomiasis and fascioliasis [60, 61, 66]. Previous reports on partial genome outline of *F. hepatica* describe an unusual genome of 10 chromosome pairs and 1.3 Gbp in size, and this duplicates and triplicates the genome size of phylogenetically related parasitic trematodes such as *Clonorchis sinensis* [547 Mbp] and *Schistosoma* spp. [398 Mbp] [28]. This excess of genomic information is considered a sample of the parasite's genetic plasticity that allows it to adapt rapidly to a changing environment, which may include the occupation of new ecological niches during the global warming process, adaptation to a wide range of hosts, and tolerance or resistance to fasciolicide treatment of the livestock.

All these possibilities may increase the future risk on public health [17]. Recently, an online database with a functional genomics query engine has been described [Trematode.net], the site hosts complete and draft genomes data of 16 trematodes species and offers unlimited

http://dx.doi.org/10.5772/intechopen.72632

Trematode	Genome size millions of base pairs	Open reading frames	GenBank available EST	GenBank available nucleotide sequences	Current status/ references
Fasciola hepatica	1275	15,740	1677	59,631	Completed/[29]
Fasciola gigantica	Uk	Uk	8397	1159	In process/[60]
Fasciolopsis buski	Uk	Uk		18	In process/[60]
Haplorchis taichui	Uk	Uk			In process/[60]
Opisthorchis felineus	Uk	Uk			In process/[60]
Paragonimus kellicotti	Uk	Uk			In process/[60]
Paragonimus miyazaki	Uk	Uk			In process/[60]
Paragonimus westermani	Uk	Uk	505	319	In process/[60]
Clonorchis sinensis	516	16,000	113,414	3401	In process/[68]
Opisthorchis viverrini	634.5	16,379	4194	101,007	Completed/[65]
Schistosoma japonicum	397	13,469	103,881	55,028	Completed/[63, 67]
Schistosoma mansoni	363	14,229	113,714	3401	Completed/[61, 64]
Schistosoma haematobium	385	11,140		4433	Completed/[62]

Uk = Unknown.

Table 5. Zoonotic trematode genome projects efforts completed and in progress. A number of genomic research institution have being working on sequencing the genomes of the most important etiological agents of zoonotic trematodiasis, the table exhibits the status of some of these projects as well as the number of estimated genes already available on line for each parasite.

downloading and online genome-transcriptome analysis tools [62]. **Table 5** depicts some information on the genomic research on zoonotic trematodes.

Author details

Estefan Miranda Miranda

Address all correspondence to: miranda.estefhan@inifap.gob.mx

National Center for Disciplinary Research in Veterinary Parasitology, National Institute for Research in Forestry Agriculture and Livestock, CENID-PAVET, INIFAP, Jiutepec, Morelos, Mexico

References

[1] Macpherson CNL. Human behaviour and the epidemiology of parasitic zoonoses. International Journal for Parasitology. 2005;**35**(11–12):1319-1331

[2] Akritidis N. Parasitic, fungal and prion zoonoses: An expanding universe of candidates for human disease. Clinical Microbiology and Infection: Official Publication of the European Society of Clinical Microbiology and Infectious Diseases. 2011;**17**(3):331-335

[3] Dimitri N. R&D incentives for neglected diseases. PLoS One. 2012;**7**(12):e50835

[4] Polley L. Navigating parasite webs and parasite flow: Emerging and re-emerging parasitic zoonoses of wildlife origin. International Journal for Parasitology. 2005;**35**(11–12): 1279-1294

[5] Report of a WHO Study Group. Control of foodborne trematode infections. World Health Organization Technical Report Series. 1995;**849**:1-157

[6] Chomel B. Control and prevention of emerging parasitic zoonoses. International Journal for Parasitology. 2008;**38**(11):1211-1217

[7] Robinson MW, Dalton JP. Zoonotic helminth infections with particular emphasis on fasciolosis and other trematodiases. Philosophical Transactions of the Royal Society B: Biological Sciences. 2009;**364**(1530):2763-2776

[8] Colwell DD, Dantas-Torres F, Otranto D. Vector-borne parasitic zoonoses: Emerging scenarios and new perspectives. Veterinary Parasitology. 2011;**182**(1):14-21

[9] Colwell R. Global climate change and infectious diseases. Emerging Infectious Diseases. 1998;**4**(3):451-452

[10] Patz JA, Graczyk TK, Geller N, Vittor AY. Effects of environmental change on emerging parasitic diseases. International Journal for Parasitology. 2000;**30**(12–13):1395-1405

[11] Fayer R. Presidential address: Global change and emerging infectious diseases. The Journal of Parasitology. 2000;**86**(6):1174-1181

[12] Dobson A. Population dynamics of pathogens with multiple host species. The American Naturalist. 2004;**164**(Suppl 5):S64-S78

[13] Sutherst RW. The vulnerability of animal and human health to parasites under global change. International Journal for Parasitology. 2001;**31**(9):933-948

[14] WHO. Climate change and human health—Risks and responses. Summary. [Internet]. WHO. Aug 29, 2016. Available from: http://www.who.int/globalchange/climate/summary/en/index5.html

[15] Thompson RCA, Kutz SJ, Smith A. Parasite zoonoses and wildlife: Emerging issues. International Journal of Environmental Research and Public Health. 2009;**6**(2):678-693

[16] Kaewkes S. Taxonomy and biology of liver flukes. Acta Tropica. 2003;**88**(3):177-186

[17] Furst T, Sayasone S, Odermatt P, Keiser J, Utzinger J. Manifestation, diagnosis, and management of foodborne trematodiasis. British Medical Journal. Jun 26, 2012;**344**(1):e4093-e4093

[18] Born-Torrijos A, Poulin R, Raga J, Holzer A. Estimating trematode prevalence in snail hosts using a single-step duplex PCR: How badly does cercarial shedding underestimate infection rates? Parasites & Vectors. 2014;**7**(1):243

[19] Lim JH, Mairiang E, Ahn GH. Biliary parasitic diseases including clonorchiasis, opisthorchiasis and fascioliasis. Abdominal Imaging. Apr 2008;**33**(2):157-165

[20] Keiser J, Utzinger J. Emerging foodborne trematodiasis. Emerging Infectious Diseases. 2005;**11**(10):1507-1514

[21] Kostadinova A. Review of "the biology of echinostomes. From the molecule to the community" by Bernard fried and Rafael Toledo [eds.]. Parasites & Vectors. 2009;**2**:52

[22] Mas-Coma S, Bargues MD, Valero MA. Fascioliasis and other plant-borne trematode zoonoses. International Journal for Parasitology. 2005;**35**(11–12):1255-1278

[23] Keiser J, Utzinger J. Food-borne trematodiases. Clinical Microbiology Reviews. 2009;**22**(3): 466-483

[24] Torgerson PR, Macpherson CNL. The socioeconomic burden of parasitic zoonoses: Global trends. Veterinary Parasitology. 2011;**182**(1):79-95

[25] Lun Z-R, Gasser RB, Lai D-H, Li A-X, Zhu X-Q, Yu X-B, et al. Clonorchiasis: A key foodborne zoonosis in China. The Lancet Infectious Diseases. 2005;**5**(1):31-41

[26] Andrews RH, Sithithaworn P, Petney TN. *Opisthorchis viverrini*: An underestimated parasite in world health. Trends in Parasitology. 2008;**24**(11):497-501

[27] Chai J-Y, Shin E-H, Lee S-H, Rim H-J. Foodborne intestinal flukes in Southeast Asia. The Korean Journal of Parasitology. 2009;**47**(Suppl):S69-S102

[28] Scarcella S, Miranda-Miranda E, Cossío-Bayúgar R, Ceballos L, Fernandez V, Solana H. Increase of carboxylesterase activity in *Fasciola hepatica* recovered from triclabendazole treated sheep. Molecular and Biochemical Parasitology. 2012;**185**(2):151-153

[29] Cwiklinski K, Dalton JP, Dufresne PJ, La Course J, Williams DJ, Hodgkinson J, et al. The *Fasciola hepatica* genome: Gene duplication and polymorphism reveals adaptation to the host environment and the capacity for rapid evolution. Genome Biology. 2015;**16**:71

[30] Fernández V, Cadenazzi G, Larsen K, Miranda-Miranda E. A Multienzyme response is involved in the phenomenon of Fasciola hepatica resistance to triclabendazole. Journal of Drug Metabolism & Toxicology [Internet]. 2015;**6**(4):1-4

[31] Zumaquero-Ríos JL, Sarracent-Pérez J, Rojas-García R, Rojas-Rivero L, Martínez-Tovilla Y, Valero MA, et al. Fascioliasis and intestinal parasitoses affecting schoolchildren in Atlixco, Puebla state, Mexico: Epidemiology and treatment with nitazoxanide. PLoS Neglected Tropical Diseases. 2013;**7**(11):e2553

[32] Koláová L, Horák P, Skírnisson K, Mareková H, Doenhoff M. Cercarial dermatitis, a neglected allergic disease. Clinical Reviews in Allergy and Immunology. 2013;**45**(1):63-74

[33] Horák P, Mike L, Lichtenbergová L, Skála V, Soldánová M, Brant SV. Avian schistosomes and outbreaks of cercarial dermatitis. Clinical Microbiology Reviews. 2015;**28**(1):165-190

[34] Brant SV, Cohen AN, James D, Hui L, Hom A, Loker ES. Cercarial dermatitis transmitted by exotic marine snail. Emerging Infectious Diseases. 2010;**16**(9):1357-1365

[35] WHO. Zoonoses and the Human-Animal-Ecosystems Interface [Internet]. Aug 29, 2016. Available from: http://www.who.int/zoonoses/en/

[36] Molyneux DH. "Neglected" diseases but unrecognised successes – Challenges and opportunities for infectious disease control. The Lancet (London, England). 2004;**364**(9431):380-383

[37] King CH, Bertino A-M. Asymmetries of poverty: Why global burden of disease valuations underestimate the burden of neglected tropical diseases. PLoS Neglected Tropical Diseases. 2008;**2**(3):e209

[38] Hotez P, Raff S, Fenwick A, Richards F, Molyneux DH. Recent progress in integrated neglected tropical disease control. Trends in Parasitology. 2007;**23**(11):511-514

[39] Hotez PJ, Molyneux DH, Fenwick A, Kumaresan J, Sachs SE, Sachs JD, et al. Control of neglected tropical diseases. The New England Journal of Medicine. 2007;**357**(10):1018-1027

[40] Hotez PJ, Brindley PJ, Bethony JM, King CH, Pearce EJ, Jacobson J. Helminth infections: The great neglected tropical diseases. The Journal of Clinical Investigation. 2008;**118**(4):1311-1321

[41] Sripa B. Concerted action is needed to tackle liver fluke infections in Asia. PLoS Neglected Tropical Diseases. 2008;**2**(5):e232

[42] Fallon PG, Doenhoff MJ. Drug-resistant schistosomiasis: Resistance to praziquantel and oxamniquine induced in *Schistosoma mansoni* in mice is drug specific. The American Journal of Tropical Medicine and Hygiene. 1994;**51**(1):83-88

[43] Devine C, Brennan GP, Lanusse CE, Alvarez LI, Trudgett A, Hoey E, et al. Piperonyl butoxide enhances triclabendazole action against triclabendazole-resistant *Fasciola hepatica*. Parasitology. 2011;**138**(2):224-236

[44] Devine C, Brennan GP, Lanusse CE, Alvarez LI, Trudgett A, Hoey E, et al. Effect of the metabolic inhibitor, methimazole on the drug susceptibility of a triclabendazole-resistant isolate of *Fasciola hepatica*. Parasitology. 2009;**136**(2):183-192

[45] Devine C, Brennan GP, Lanusse CE, Alvarez LI, Trudgett A, Hoey E, et al. Inhibition of cytochrome P450-mediated metabolism enhances ex vivo susceptibility of *Fasciola hepatica* to triclabendazole. Parasitology. 2010;**137**(5):871-880

[46] Virkel G, Lifschitz A, Sallovitz J, Pis A, Lanusse C. Assessment of the main metabolism pathways for the flukicidal compound triclabendazole in sheep. Journal of Veterinary Pharmacology and Therapeutics. 2006;**29**(3):213-223

[47] Young ND, Hall RS, Jex AR, Cantacessi C, Gasser RB. Elucidating the transcriptome of *Fasciola hepatica*—A key to fundamental and biotechnological discoveries for a neglected parasite. Biotechnology Advances 2010;**28**(2):222-231

[48] Calvopiña M, Cevallos W, Kumazawa H, Eisenberg J. High prevalence of human liver infection by *Amphimerus* spp. flukes, Ecuador. Emerging Infectious Diseases. 2011;**17**(12): 2331-2334

[49] i-xvi—ZoonosesVol-3.pdf [Internet]. Aug 30, 2016. Available from: http://www1.paho.org/hq/dmdocuments/2010/ZoonosesVol-3.pdf

[50] WHO. Preventive Chemotherapy in Human Helminthiasis [Internet]. Aug 29, 2016. Available from: http://www.who.int/neglected_diseases/preventive_chemotherapy/pct_manual/en/

[51] Johansen MV, Lier T, Sithithaworn P. Towards improved diagnosis of neglected zoonotic trematodes using a one health approach. Acta Tropica. 2015;**141**:161-169

[52] Mazeri S, Sargison N, Kelly RF, Bronsvoort BM de C, Handel I. Evaluation of the performance of five diagnostic tests for *Fasciola hepatica* infection in naturally infected cattle using a Bayesian no gold standard approach. PLoS One. 2016;**11**(8):e0161621

[53] Adela Valero M, Victoria Periago M, Pérez-Crespo I, Rodríguez E, Jesús Perteguer M, Gárate T, et al. Assessing the validity of an ELISA test for the serological diagnosis of human fascioliasis in different epidemiological situations: Assessing the validity of an ELISA test. Tropical Medicine & International Health. 2012;**17**(5):630-636

[54] Kajugu P-E, Hanna REB, Edgar HW, McMahon C, Cooper M, Gordon A, et al. *Fasciola hepatica*: Specificity of a coproantigen ELISA test for diagnosis of fasciolosis in faecal samples from cattle and sheep concurrently infected with gastrointestinal nematodes, coccidians and/or rumen flukes [paramphistomes], under field conditions. Veterinary Parasitology. 2015;**212**(3–4):181-187

[55] Khandelwal N, Shaw J, Jain MK. Biliary parasites: Diagnostic and therapeutic strategies. Current Treatment Options in Gastroenterology. 2008;**11**(2):85-95

[56] Estuningsih E, Spithill T, Raadsma H, Law R, Adiwinata G, Meeusen E, et al. Development and application of a fecal antigen diagnostic sandwich ELISA for estimating prevalence of *Fasciola gigantica* in cattle in central java, Indonesia. The Journal of Parasitology. 2009;**95**(2):450-455

[57] Córdova M, Reátegui L, Espinoza JR. Immunodiagnosis of human fascioliasis with *Fasciola hepatica* cysteine proteinases. Transactions of the Royal Society of Tropical Medicine and Hygiene. 1999;**93**(1):54-57

[58] Duenngai K, Sithithaworn P, Rudrappa UK, Iddya K, Laha T, Stensvold CR, et al. Improvement of PCR for detection of *Opisthorchis viverrini* DNA in human stool samples. Journal of Clinical Microbiology. 2008;**46**(1):366-368

[59] Cnops L, Tannich E, Polman K, Clerinx J, Van Esbroeck M. Schistosoma real-time PCR as diagnostic tool for international travellers and migrants: Schistosoma real-time PCR as diagnostic tool. Tropical Medicine & International Health. 2012;**17**(10):1208-1216

[60] Martin J, Rosa BA, Ozersky P, Hallsworth-Pepin K, Zhang X, Bhonagiri-Palsikar V, et al. Helminth.net: Expansions to Nematode.net and an introduction to Trematode.net. Nucleic Acids Research. 2015;**43**(D1):D698-D706

[61] Protasio AV, Tsai IJ, Babbage A, Nichol S, Hunt M, Aslett MA, et al. A systematically improved high quality genome and transcriptome of the human blood fluke *Schistosoma mansoni*. PLoS Neglected Tropical Diseases. 2012;**6**(1):e1455

[62] Young ND, Jex AR, Li B, Liu S, Yang L, Xiong Z, et al. Whole-genome sequence of *Schistosoma haematobium*. Nature Genetics. 2012;**44**(2):221-225

[63] Zhou Y, Zheng H, Chen Y, Zhang L, Wang K, Guo J, et al. The *Schistosoma japonicum* genome reveals features of host–parasite interplay. Nature. 2009;**460**(7253):345-351

[64] Oliveira G, Franco G, Verjovski-Almeida S. The Brazilian contribution to the study of the *Schistosoma mansoni* transcriptome. Acta Tropica. 2008;**108**(2–3):179-182

[65] Young ND, Nagarajan N, Lin SJ, Korhonen PK, Jex AR, Hall RS, et al. The Opisthorchis viverrini genome provides insights into life in the bile duct. Nature Communications [Internet]. 2014;**5**:1-11

[66] McGonigle L, Mousley A, Marks NJ, Brennan GP, Dalton JP, Spithill TW, et al. The silencing of cysteine proteases in *Fasciola hepatica* newly excysted juveniles using RNA interference reduces gut penetration. International Journal for Parasitology. 2008;**38**(2):149-155

[67] Xue X, Sun J, Zhang Q, Wang Z, Huang Y, Pan W. Identification and Characterization of Novel MicroRNAs from *Schistosoma japonicum*. Carlow CKS, editor. PLoS ONE. 2008;**3**(12): e4034

[68] Wang X, Chen W, Huang Y, Sun J, Men J, Liu H, et al. The draft genome of the carcinogenic human liver fluke *Clonorchis sinensis*. Genome Biology. 2011;**12**(10):R107

Chapter 10

Metagenomics and Diagnosis of Zoonotic Diseases

Laura Inés Cuervo-Soto,
Silvio Alejandro López-Pazos and
Ramón Alberto Batista-García

Additional information is available at the end of the chapter

http://dx.doi.org/10.5772/intechopen.72634

Abstract

Zoonotic diseases represent a public health problem worldwide, since approximately 60% of human pathogens have a zoonotic origin. A variety of methodologies have been developed to diagnose zoonosis, including culture-dependent and immunological-based methods, which allow the identification of a huge range of pathogens. However, some of them are not detected easily with these approaches. Additionally, molecular tests have been developed, and they are designed to identify a single pathogen or mixtures of them. In this context, metagenomics comes as an alternative to get genome sequences of different microorganisms, which comprise a microbial community. Metagenomics have been used to characterize microbiomes and viromes, which are not cultivable under laboratory conditions. This methodology could be a powerful tool in the diagnosis of zoonotic diseases because it allows not only identification of genus and species, but also detection of some proteins in specific conditions on specific tissues, through structural and functional metagenomics, respectively.

Keywords: zoonosis, metagenomics, virome, microbiome, diagnostic

1. Introduction

Zoonotic diseases represent a public health problem worldwide, since approximately 60% of human pathogens have a zoonotic origin. Many of the most important human pathogens are either zoonotic or originated as zoonosis before adapting to humans. Consequently, humans are continuously being exposed to novel animal pathogens [1, 2].

In recent years, the epidemiological safety has been threatened with new emerging zoonotic diseases such as Zika, Ebola, H1N1 influenza and severe acute respiratory syndrome. Several risk assessment studies have estimated that 75% of emerging pathogens are zoonotic in origin (OPS 2016). The rise of these emerging diseases might be related to the increase in population, the growth of cities, the destruction of natural habitats, the modernization of agricultural practices and the climate change, among others [3, 4].

Zoonotic diseases are pathologies that can be distributed between animals and humans. Fungi, parasites, bacterias and viruses, being bacteria and viruses the zoonotic agents more prevalent can cause different zoonosis are very common and have a high frequency in the population. They are derived from the interactions with animals during the daily activities. Taylor and coworkers reported that of 1415 pathogens known to infect humans, 61% were or are zoonotic [5].

Animals are important elements in our daily lives. They inhabit our houses, some as pets; we have a close contact with them in the zoo; animals are essential part of the agricultural practices around the world. The saliva, blood, urine or feces of animals, which are infected, transmit zoonotic agents. Several animals are only carrier of different pathogens for human, but they do not develop the illness. These animals are defined as vector. Probably, the most famous vector is the mosquito *Aedes aegypti*. This mosquito is the causal agent of dengue, an important viral disease in tropical zones in America, Africa and Asia. Another way to get a zoonotic disease is through food consumption. It is very frequent in our countries to consume unpasteurized milk, undercooked meat or fish, unwashed fruits and vegetables, which can be contaminated with urine and feces from infected animals. Zoonoses can be dangerous, and some of them can cause death if not diagnosed and treated on time. Thus, zoonotic can be acquired if we work with animals, have pets, practice hobbies involving animals or consume water or food contaminated with pathogens from animals.

The World Organization for Health recognizes as the most common zoonotic disease as:

1. Lyme disease and Rocky Mountain spotted fever, both transmitted by a tick bite.

2. West Nile virus (WNV) transmitted by a mosquito bite.

3. Dengue, malaria and chikungunya transmitted by an infected mosquito.

4. *Salmonella* infections transmitted by baby chick, chicken, duck, turtle or snake.

5. *Escherichia coli* infections transmitted by infected animals, such as cows.

With this in mind, zoonoses are a considerable risk to human health. Derived of this, important research projects are being developed to understand and study the epidemiology, dynamics, distribution and infection of zoonotic agents. However, the diagnosis of zoonotic agents, and the description and distribution of new zoonotic microorganisms and viruses remain a challenge for international public health. Therefore, the study of the microbiota of free-living animals as well as pets provides useful knowledge for prediction and treatment of new zoonoses. Different areas of knowledge are included in this purpose, such as molecular biology, immunology and epidemiology, among others.

2. Conventional diagnosis

A variety of methodologies have been developed to diagnose zoonoses. For example, the culture of microorganisms allows the easy identification of a huge range of pathogens. However, some of them are not detected easily with this approach. In this case, these microorganisms are underestimated or frequently misdiagnosed. Some of them are predominant and can be highly prevalent and important in the environment. Parallel with the culture methods, microscopy techniques to identify pathogens from tissues have provided an important support in the diagnosis of zoonotic diseases. The sampling of some tissues is usually very invasive, this being an important disadvantage. These approaches are complementary.

Important advances in the diagnosis of zoonotic diseases have been achieved over time. Various antigen-based assays and methods are used for the diagnosis of these diseases, optimizing handling and security of samples and decreasing the time in reporting the results. Serological assays are used for the detection of antibodies in serum samples from humans. Indirect fluorescent antibody (IFA), indirect hemagglutination assay, complement fixation, direct agglutination test (DAT) and enzyme-linked immunosorbent assay (ELISA) are some of these assays with different specificities and sensitivities [6, 7]. But up to date, the antibody availability is a huge problem. The pathogen classification considering several serotypes and other pathogenic characteristics is limited to the existence of specific antibodies.

The development of test such as Western blotting and immunochromatographic test using antigens produced by genetic engineering have enabled the confirmation of serological tests to differentiate strains within a species and identify some virulence factors involved in the pathogenic disease process. Given the new developments at the genomic level from the 50s, several technologies for nucleic acid manipulation of infectious agents have been developed, such as the polymerase chain reaction (PCR), restriction fragment length polymorphism (RFLP), pulse field gel electrophoresis (PFGE), random amplified polymorphic DNA (RAPD), ribotyping, spoligotyping, high-throughput sequencing and qPCR for use in clinical samples from humans and animals. These techniques have been successfully used to diagnose animal pathogens. Although molecular methods provide high specificity and sensitivity, they have been used mainly in research studies and not in clinical diagnosis. Their expensive costs can explain the above. The molecular diagnosis is designed to identify a single pathogen or mixtures of them, but considering a limited number of them. This scope is very simple if we want to study the microbial interactions between pathogens and the resident microbiota in any organism. It is known that these interactions are epidemiologically very important and can influence in the illness [8]. Thus, it is essential to develop new methodologies capable to detect simultaneously multiple pathogens and allow to take in context with the resident microbiota. With this in mind, the clinical diagnosis demands new approaches to study the presence of any pathogens and, at the same time, their interaction with other microorganisms, microbial populations and communities.

Particularly, viruses are the most abundant form of life on the Earth. However, few groups of them can be cultivated in laboratory conditions. They can be identified using several methods, such as electron microscopy, cell culture, inoculation and serology, among others. All these techniques require a previous knowledge of the virus because they are based on comparisons with known viruses. Those viruses that cannot be cultivated in the laboratory can be identified by molecular methods such as microarray, subtractive hybridization-based and PCR-based methods [9]. To apply molecular methods to characterize viruses also requires previous information about the target virus. However, some new methods have overcome this limitation: sequence-independent single primer amplification, degenerate oligonucleotide primed

PCR, random PCR and rolling circle amplification [9]. But, all these techniques do not allow the complete understanding of the virome in both animals and humans.

Next-generation sequencing (NGS) techniques are definitively new tools to get a complete understanding of the viral composition in humans and animals. These sequencing tools have many applications in research and diagnosis in humans and animals, and they are allowing the high-throughput prospections to identify pathogen viruses in animals [10]. Next-generation sequencing techniques offer thousands to millions of reads able to detect any virus in few copies. Thus, global studies to prospect the viral composition of any organism are necessary to advance in our understanding of zoonoses.

3. Metagenomics as a diagnostic tool

Metagenomics is an alternative to get genome sequences from differents microbial community. This approach have been used with diagnostic proposes (**Figure 1**). Metagenomics-based approaches have over the past few decades been developed in efforts to assess, analyze and exploit biodiversity in a wide variety of different environmental niches. Metagenomics approaches have gained importance in clinical studies, even with diagnostic proposes. Conventional diagnostic (cultivation-dependent methods) identifies pathogen species, strains and serotypes of interest in independent colonies through isolation of microorganisms and obtaining axenic cultures. For this reason, diagnostic investigation of pathogen microbes through culture-independent methods has become invaluable, with metagenomics being employed to study microbiomes and viromes, which are not cultivable under laboratory conditions.

There are two main areas in metagenomics: structural and functional metagenomics. The first of them is relevant to analyze, identify and describe the microbiomes and viromes in animals and humans. Structural metagenomics studies the composition of microbial populations and communities describing the major genera and species that colonize tissues or

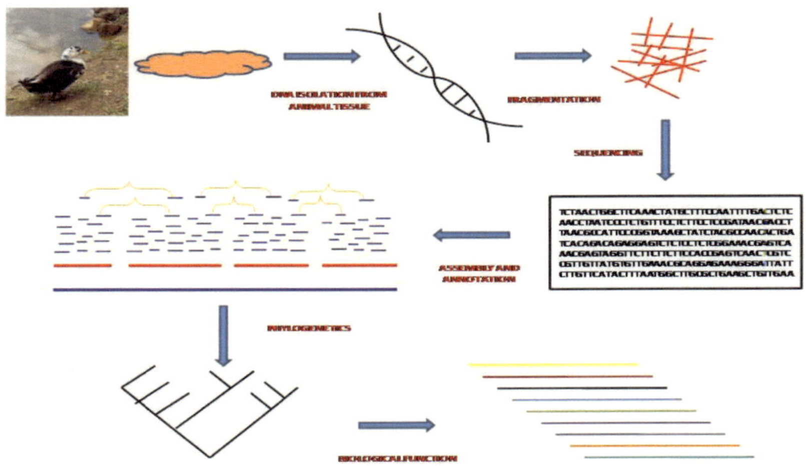

Figure 1. Metagenomics for zoonotic diseases.

organisms. It also provides relevant information about the ecological niches of microorganisms and hypothesizes about relationships established between pathogens, hosts and native microbiomes/viromes.

On the other hand, functional metagenomic would be attractive in the diagnostic field, since some proteins would be detected in specific conditions on specific tissues. The best contribution to knowledge of the structural metagenomic approach has been to identify truly novel species and genera. Some of these have no close relatives and even form deeply branched lineages.

The extraction of high-quality DNA is the first critical step in the metagenomic analysis. Frequently, a huge quantity of human or animal DNA is isolated when microbiomes and viromes are studied from humans or animal samples. This approach was originally developed to analyze microbial genomes contained in environmental samples, but in the last decade its application has been extended to describe new animal and human pathogens. Also, metagenomics has been used to characterize microbiomes and viromes from different tissues and organisms, being relevant in clinical microbiology with a great impact on public health [2, 11]. Other global studies are also important to study animal pathogens, such as metatranscriptomics, metaproteomics and lipidomics, among others. The high-throughput sequencing technologies allow getting a huge sequence database including genes, transcripts and proteins and also allow establishing metabolic networks to understand the relationship between pathogens and hosts [11, 12].

Microorganisms colonize a wide variety of hosts, including animal and humans. They have very specialized ecological niches, even colonize and sicken tissues and whole organisms. Prokaryotic organisms show the highest metabolic diversity and they have been extensively studied as animal pathogens. Viruses are the most abundant in the nature and they are considered as important zoonotic agents.

Metagenomics and high-throughput sequencing technologies are allowing an increase of the studies related to zoonotic diseases and microbiota in animals. These technologies generate millions of short sequence reads (approximately 150 pb) and facilitate the analysis, since cloning procedures are not required. Metagenomics is a powerful and useful tool to describe the diversity and dynamic of bacteria, virus and fungal species in tissues and samples obtained from different animals.

In addition to the findings of viral genomes, metagenomics has contributed to the characterization of microbiomes in different samples, such as canine oral cavity healthy dogs and gastrointestinal tract of several organisms (e.g., feline, canine, human, mouse and chicken). These studies have found taxonomic units with zoonotic potentialities. On the other hand, the previous works revealed a closely phylogenetic relationship between microbiomes from different organisms [13, 14].

Infectious viral diseases, both emerging and reemerging, remain a threat to human and animal health. The increase in these infections appears to be related to human activities and climatic changes which cause outbreaks and pandemics. Some viruses related to these outbreaks are the influenza A viruses, Ebola, Middle East Respiratory Syndrome (MERS) coronavirus and new viruses belonging to the family Bunyaviridae, as the Schmallenberg virus. It is possible that Ebola virus was introduced into the human population through zoonotic transmission by fruit bat (*Pteripodidae*). It is known that Schmallenberg virus was the agent of outbreaks in ruminants in the European Union. The virus was propagated from the Middle East to the Republic of Korea, causing 186 confirmed human cases with 36 deaths in July 2015 [2]. Moreover, zoonotic viruses, bacteria and parasites can be transmitted to humans from livestock production chain or wild animals, which are used as food (e.g., domestic vertebrates and invertebrates). This situation represents a serious infection risk for humans. The infection transmission and its amplification in the population may occur when the causative agents in wildlife are mobilized and introduced into new hosts like cattle, causing outbreaks that amplify the pathogen transmission to humans [1].

3.1. Metagenomics for viral diagnostics?

Viral metagenomics is a culture-independent approach that is used to investigate the complete viral genetic populations of a biological sample. This methodology becomes a powerful tool for identifying new and emerging viruses, considering that animals remain a reservoir for the virus that can cause zoonosis. Increased knowledge of the viral flora in healthy and diseased individuals is important for both animal and human health [15]. In this regard, the metagenomic assays for the discovery of viruses are based mainly on the sequence-independent amplification of nucleic acids from clinical samples, in combination with next-generation sequencing platforms and bioinformatics tools for sequence analysis. They are relatively simple and fast and allow detection of hundreds of viruses simultaneously, even unknown viruses that might be highly divergent from those that are already described [2]. These platforms offer different throughputs, as mentioned by [15]. High-throughput sequencing technology, Roche 454, is based on pyrosequencing; its throughput is 0.4–0.6 Gb/run, with reads of 400 nt. Solexa/Illumina uses a system with reversible terminators and has a higher throughput (7.5 Gb–1.8 Tb/run) with a read length of 75–150 nt depending on the sequencing system. SOLiD system is based on ligation and cleavable probes; its throughput is 80–320 Gb/run, but it produces reads of only 50–75 nt, making sequence analysis more difficult. These technologies have allowed the detection of new and known viruses from diverse samples such as animal tissues (e.g., brain, lymph nodes), insects (bees), fecal stools and oral swabs. Identified viruses by this approach are among astrovirus, bornavirus, tornovirus i, circovirustipo 2, parvovirus, coronavirus and herpesvirus [15].

In addition, some protocols for the detection, purification and enrichment of virus from organ tissue have also been developed. Kohl and coworkers proposed a method called tissue-based universal virus detection for viral metagenomics (TUViD-VM) [16]. This approach was used in chicken tissues inoculated with one of four viruses: poxvirus (vaccinia virus) representing DNA virus with envelope, Reovirus (Orthoreovirus) nonenveloped viruses, orthomyxoviruses (influenza viruses), paramyxoviruses (Sendai virus) and RNA enveloped viruses. Viruses were specially selected for their potential to cause viral emerging diseases. The developed protocol considers several steps as tissue homogenization, ultracentrifugation for the separation of viral particles, RNA extraction, amplification and finally random next-generation sequencing (NGS). The established protocol allowed the quick and reliable purification and enrichment of virus, and an increase in the amount of detectable viral nucleic acids with a sensitivity of 100–1000 virus copies/mL of homogenized organ material. This TUViD-VM protocol can be used in metagenomic and virome studies to increase the likelihood of detecting viruses from any biological source (**Figure 2**).

A workflow was developed for recuperation of complete genomes of new virions from metagenome projects. Several phases were considered, starting with the assembly of the reads into long fragments with assignment of specific contigs (named seed) from the desired virus. The analysis can then continue in linkage of other fragments to the seed contig to raise a tentative genome. Finally, a full-length viral genome is obtained (**Figure 3**).

Metagenomics is a relevant method in identification of virus causing gastrointestinal diseases in animals. Several viromes have been studied by metagenomics approaches, which have been related to zoonosis. For example, it has been reported that horses have different phages, such as *Siphoviridae, Myoviridae* and *Podoviridae.* These viral particles can control bacterial populations inhabiting into the gastrointestinal tract. On the other hand, pigs contain viral sequences corresponding to kobuviruses, enteroviruses, sapeloviruses, teschoviruses, sapoviruses, astroviruses, coronaviruses, also the families *Circoviridae* and *Parvoviridae,* and bocaviruses and posavirus 1 and 2 (RNA virus). Some of them have been related to illness in different animals. Additionally, a described case in rabbit revealed a great number of Astrovirus sequences related to enteric disease. Other study reported in diarrheic dogs, the presence of canine parvovirus 2 (CPV2), canine enteric coronavirus (CcoV), rotavirus, insect and plant viruses, canine kobuviruses and sapoviruses (canine sapovirus 1 and 2). Finally, studies from bird feces (turkey and chicken with enteric disease) showed kobuviruses, calicivirus (*Sapovirus* and *Lagovirus*), avianastrovirus and avian reovirus [17].

Metagenomics profiles have exhaustively allowed to know the associated arboviruses to the principal hematophagous arthropods with medical importance. *Flaviviridae* (TBEV, OHFV, SREV and WNV), *Bunyaviridae* (KKV, CCHFV and SOLV), *Reoviridae* (CTFV), *Hepadnaviridae* (HBV), *Rhabdoviridae* and *Togoviridae* (CHIKV and ONNV) are viruses detected in blood-feeding

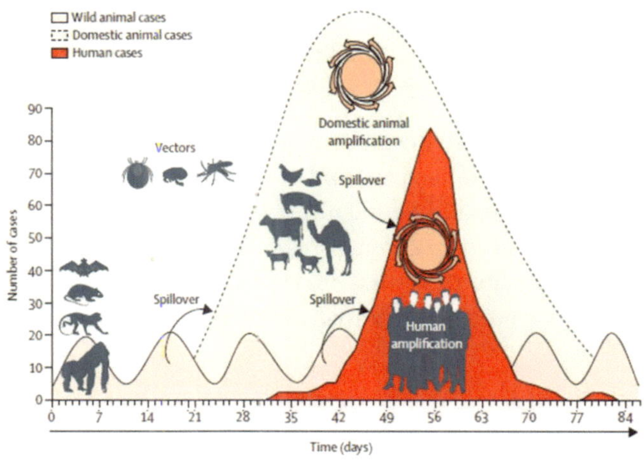

Figure 2. Clinical relevance of disease ecology. Transmission of infection and amplification in people (bright red) occurs after a pathogen from wild animals (pink) moves into livestock to cause an outbreak (light green) that amplifies the capacity for pathogen transmission to people (figure and legend were taken from [1]).

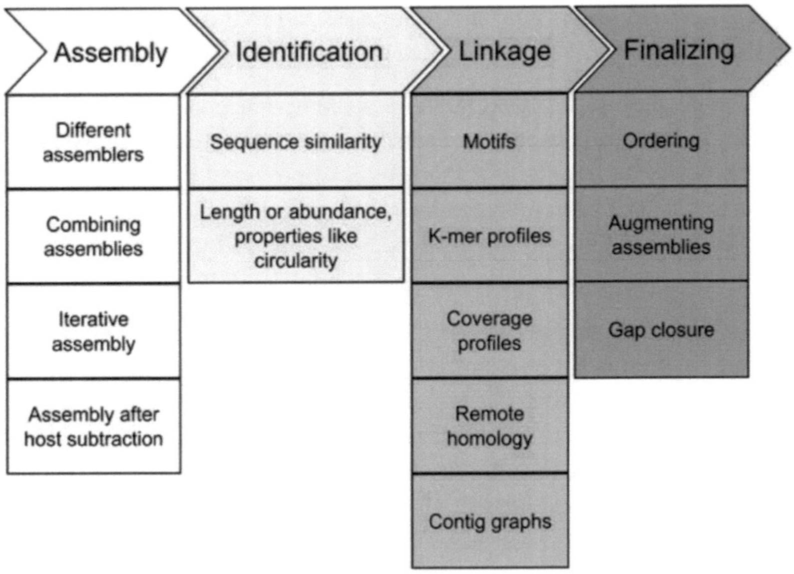

Figure 3. Steps in recovery of full-length viral genomes from metagenomes. Figure and legend were taken with permission from [2]. http://www.frontiersin.org/files/Articles/165597/fmicb-06-01069-HTML/image_m/fmicb-06-01069-g003.jpg.

arthropods by serological or molecular techniques [18]. Metagenomic studies have found animal viruses in mosquitoes, which can infect to human and/or transmit zoonosis. *Anelloviridae, Circoviridae, Herpesviridae, Poxviridae* and *Papillomaviridae* have been detected in mixed-species female mosquitoes [19]. In other arthropod species as *Anopheles* sp., *Ochlerotatus* sp., *Culex* sp. and *Aedes* sp., several animal viruses are reported: *Reoviridae (Orbivirus), Rhabdoviridae, Bunyaviridae, Flaviviridae* and *Togaviridae* [20–22]. The virome of arthropods is very important because humans and arthropods share a common habitat and they cause serious diseases, even epidemic. Metagenomic has revealed a large number of known and unknown insect-specific or zoonotic agents associated with arthropods [23, 24]. RNA virome of arthropods is under study; however, mosquitoes largely transmit RNA viruses.

Metagenomic studies conducted in mosquitoes in Australia revealed the presence of animal viruses as Edge Hill virus and Walla virus, and other virus able to infect marsupials [20]. In the same metagenomic profile could be identified viruses that infect humans, such as Ross River virus and *Alphavirus*. *Alphavirus* belongs to the *Togaviridae* family, and it is the main etiologic agent in Australia of the influenza-like illness and/or polyarthritis [20]. In this metagenomic study has also reported a novel virus, a dipteran-mammal-associated rhabdovirus: dimarhadbovirus.

These new methodologies that increase the ability to detect different species of viruses are of great interest in the diagnosis of many zoonoses. New adenoviruses have been discovered over the past 3 years, and some have been implicated as pathogens for humans. These findings show that many viruses of this kind can be discovered in the future. The detection of these viruses from rodent samples, its main host, would establish control measures to prevent or reduce the proportion of zoonotic diseases caused by them, whose manifestations in

http://dx.doi.org/10.5772/intechopen.72634

humans are known to cause a severe hemorrhagic fever, acute central nervous system disease, congenital malformations, and infection in organ transplantation recipients [25].

Other important advances in determining viruses have been shown by Dacheux and coworkers. In this study using some above-mentioned technologies, they determined the viral diversity of five different species of insectivorous bats French, who are in close contact with humans. The viromes described in this work revealed the presence of families of known viruses that infect bacteria, plants/fungi, insects or vertebrates. The most relevant groups were those that potentially infect mammals (e.g., Retroviridae, Herpesviridae, Bunyaviridae, Poxviridae, Flaviviridae, Reoviridae, Bornaviridae and Picobirnaviridae). The data revealed the detection of new viruses of mammals, including rotaviruses, gammaretroviruses, bornaviruses and bunyaviruses with the identification of the first bat nairovirus (**Figure 4**) [26].

These findings are of great interest because they demonstrated that bats naturally harbor viruses, which can infect mammals. The identification of known and unknown viruses in these natural hosts also allows to determine the role played by bats in the spread of zoonotic viral infections [26].

The first evidence of viral metagenomics was published by Breitbart et al. [27]. In this chapter, authors concluded that the viral diversity has been totally underestimated. Viruses are considered as the most abundant and diverse form of life in the nature [28], with more than 7000 different viral genotypes found in the marine ecosystems. Viral metagenomics has studied the viral composition associated with different body sites, and DNA virus communities are the mainly studied [29]. Viral metagenomic approaches in animals bring the opportunity to describe novel antibiotic resistance genes, new virulence factors and new genotypes in specific animal species [30]. For example, it surely recovers novel anellovirus sequences from animal as have been found from blood samples in humans [29].

On the other hand, bacteriophages are ubiquitously and widely distributed in any ecosystem, with estimation between 10^{13} and 10^{15} particles in the human body [31].

For example, several works have reported bacteriophage populations in salivary [32], respiratory tract [33], gastrointestinal tract [34] and oropharyngeal samples [35]. It is known that viruses of bacteria play an important role on the dynamic of bacteria populations in human

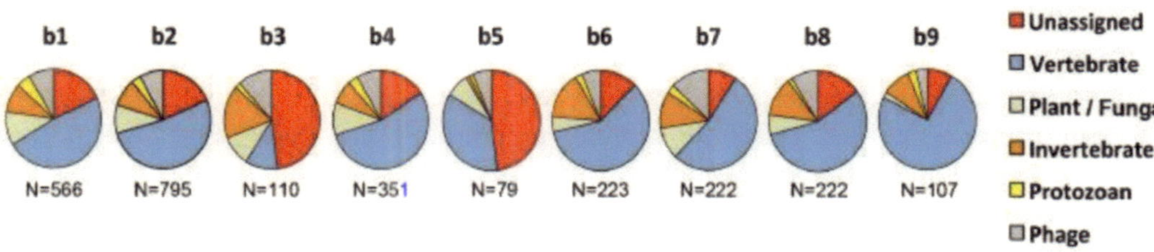

Figure 4. Distribution of contig sequences after BLASTx analysis. Percentage of sequences related to the main categories of existing viruses: vertebrate (blue), plant/fungal (green), invertebrate (brown), protozoan (yellow) viruses and bacteriophages (gray), and unassigned viral sequences (no data available concerning the taxonomic family, indicated in red). The total number of viral contigs is indicated below each pie chart (figure and legend were taken with permission from [17]). http://journals.plos.org/plosone/article?id=10.1371/journal.pone.0087194.

and have influence on the horizontal gene transfer processes, among others [36, 37]. In this sense, Breitbart and Rohwer in 2005 published that bacteriophages can also play important roles on healthy and disease states in humans. They can confer new pathogenic phenotype in pathogenic bacteria. To study this phenomenon in animals can be interesting because we allow to develop new diagnostic assays, identify new pathogenic factors and design new therapies for zoonosis. Metagenomic profiles of viral compositions have suggested that the human oropharynx is an important reservoir of virulence genes [33]. There are strong evidences of horizontal gene transfer from bacteriophages to bacteria in humans, because antibiotic resistance genes have been found in bacteriophages studied in cystic fibrosis patients [38]. These studies not only allow to identify the viral composition in humans and animals, but also allow to confirm the presence of known and unknown virulence genes, the dynamic between viruses and bacteria and design new diagnostic tools.

Metagenomic approaches have been successfully used to study emergent viruses. These global tools were applied to study the yellow fever virus in the hemorrhagic fever in Uganda and the flu virus, both in 2010. Metagenomics allowed to elucidate the complete genome of the flu virus, when the information about this virus was totally missing [39, 40]. Thus, metagenomics has important implications to study new emergent virus and its genome and consequently take in advance controls to prevent their dissemination. The results obtained from metagenomic studies in humans and animals have also positive impact in the development of new and robust molecular techniques with diagnostic interest.

The collection of a good and representative sample is necessary with metagenomic proposes. Viral enriched sample can be obtained by filtration and ultracentrifugation, and particles are purified with sucrose, glycerol or cesium chloride density gradient [41]. Because viral genome is shorter than those in prokaryotic and eukaryotic cells, the filtration is essential to remove bacteria and host cells. However, if we use filters of 0.2 μm, large viruses are totally missing in the sample and the viral fingerprinting will be underestimated. So, methodological details should be adjusted with our particular interest.

The amplification of viral genome is usually recommended before nucleic acid extractions. Linker amplified shotgun library method is frequently used to amplify viral genomes. Viral DNA or cDNA obtained from RNA viruses should be fragmented, ligated and PCR-amplified [27]. But this technique has an important disadvantage because ssDNA viral genomes cannot be amplified and they are missing in the final metagenome [42]. The isothermal amplification of the DNA or cDNA obtained from RNA viruses is also recommended by using random hexamer and the phi29 DNA polymerase. This methodology is called multiple displacement amplification, and it is an alternative technique to linker amplified shotgun library method. Multiple displacement amplification is preferentially used to amplify ssDNA [42, 43]. It is important to note that the used amplification method will have a significant influence on the metagenome preparation and consequently on downstream analyses and comparisons.

After metagenome preparation, a bioinformatics workflow is necessary to make good and accurate interpretations. This workflow includes in general four steps: preprocessing, annotation, assembly and, finally, the estimation of genotypes, abundances, community, structure and diversity. During the annotation, several databases are specifically used for viruses, such as ProVide [44], MGTAXA [http://mgtaxa.jcvi.org], MetaVir [45], VIROME [Bhavsar et al. in preparation] and VMGAP [46].

The taxonomic classification is defined as an active field in viral metagenomics [30]. Two main methods are used to classify the sequence with taxonomic proposes: similarity-based methods and composition-based methods.

Viral metagenomics has really allowed us to describe pathogen viral agents for diverse diseases [10, 15, 47–49]. Metagenomic tools have also conducted to characterize the baseline viral diversity for humans and animals [18].

3.2. Bacterial metagenomics

Bacteria are an important microbial group that frequently causes zoonosis. Many bacteria are zoonotic agents involved in gastrointestinal diseases, which affect a wide group of animals. An important microbiome is contained inside the gastrointestinal tract of animals as a proof of selection process of microbes by host gut and specific feed. Complete knowledge about gastrointestinal tract microbiome is not possible with conventional culture, but metagenomics supports a great amount of biological data that reflect the gastrointestinal tract microorganisms and their potential [50, 51]. For example, *Campylobacter jejuni* colonizes the ceca of chickens without causing disease approximately at 3 weeks of age and this remains present throughout the chicken life.

A metagenomics analysis of chicken cecal microbiome using both free-pathogen and *C. jejuni*-infected individuals revealed a high distribution of *Actinobacteria, Bacteroides, Chlorobi, Deferribacteres, Firmicutes, Fusobacteria, Proteobacteria* and *Verrucomicrobia. Firmicutes* is the most important phylla independent of chicken type, and it was dominant in all chicken ceca. *Bacteriodes* phylla had high abundance in free-pathogen chicken. *Campylobacter*-like sequences were found in the chicken infected with *C. jejuni*. There were not identified archaea sequences, and some Eukarya sequences were determined in this study [52].

The metagenomic has allowed the description of microbiomes from samples obtained of a limited number of mammalian species. The study of microbiome from wild and domestic animals brings an important knowledge about resident and pathogen microorganisms that can be transmitted to the human and to cause several diseases. For example, there is an increase interest to study the bat-associated microbiota because bats are an important reservoir and vector of zoonotic pathogens [53]. Bats are widely distributed in the world, being the second diversity species of mammals [54]. They inhabit forests, gardens, orchards and agricultural areas, among other ecosystems. Thus, it is very important as zoonotic control to know the microbiome in bat, particularly pathogenic bacteria and viruses [53]. Some previous studies focused on virus have reported the presence of Rabies virus [55], Nipah virus [56, 57], Hendra virus [58], and European and Australian bat lyssaviruses [59], among others. We have to note that the study of pathogenic bacteria in bats has been poorly considered. Few works have reported the presence of *Salmonella* spp. [60] and *Clostridium* spp. [61] isolated from bat samples.

The metagenomics brings new possibilities to describe extensively the pathogenic microbiota inhabiting in bats since culture-based methods are very limited. Hatta and coworkers studied the rectal microbiota in bats using high-throughput sequencing of V3-V4 region of the 16S rRNA. They found the presence of 103 genera of bacteria. *Campylobacter* was detected as a prevalent genus being identified *C. jejuni* and *C. coli* in rectal samples from bits (*Rousettus amplexicaudatus*). *C. jejuni* is defined as a serious agent for diarrheic diseases in humans, and bats are an important reservoir for this species. This study revealed that the predominant phyla was Firmicutes, and the authors identified 66 families, *Clostridiaceae, Campylobacteraceae* and *Enterobacteriaceae* as being predominant. Moreover, 103 genera were classified and *Clostridium* and *Campylobacter* were the majority. Other studies have described as dominant genera to *Leuconostoc, Betaproteobacteria* and *Enterobacter*.

Brucellosis is other zoonosis extensively found in humans, causing 500,000 human infections per year around the world. *Brucella melitensis* affects humans through consumption of infected milk, meat or animal contact, leading to spreading into reticuloendothelial tissue or osteoarticular effects. Shotgun metagenomics is a useful option to detect Brucellosis in historical human material. A study on a skeleton of a ~60-year-old male with features of diffuse idiopathic skeletal hyperostosis and 32 calcified nodules in the pelvic girdle was carried up in order to identify *Brucella*'s sequences. It was obtained 10,000 sequences related with *B. melitensis* genomes, providing approximately 0.7-fold coverage of a medieval *Brucella* genome from the strain Geridu-1. Sequences showed abundant CT and GA base conversions, a signal of the damage in ancient DNA. A phylogenetic analysis provides evidences that the *B. melitensis* Geridu-1 is closely connected with four *B. melitensis* strains. Additional tests such as deletions and locations of insertion sequences confirm the assignment of the Geridu-1 strain within *B. melitensis* [62].

Many studies have been performed to describe the oral flora in dogs and cats, since these animals are very frequently found as pets. Microorganisms, especially the bacteria in the oral cavity, play important physiological roles. They provide protection against opportunist pathogens and are an essential barrier with the host immune system [63]. But, the oral flora also can cause dental caries, periodontitis and systemic infections, among others [64]. Considering that dogs are the most common companion animals, Oh and coworkers published a work describing the composition of the canine oral microbiome [65]. They found in the dog's microbiome human pathogen bacteria, and at the same time, the authors concluded that its relationships with the owners are largely unclear. In this study, 246 operational taxonomic units were detected in 10 samples from dogs and their owners, where Firmicutes, Proteobacteria, Bacteroidetes, Fusobacteria and Actinobacteria were the predominant phyla in human oral cavity. On the other hand, Proteobacteria, Actinobacteria, Bacteroidetes, Firmicutes and Fusobacteria were predominant in oral sample of the sampled dogs. Related studies have been developed in order to clarify and understand the dynamic of oral-to-oral transfer of zoonotic bacteria. Oh and coworkers concluded that the oral microbiomes of dogs and their owners were different. Regarding the oral-to-oral transfer, the authors recovered evidence that *Neisseria shayeganii, Porphyromonas canigingivalis, Tannerella forsythia* and *Streptococcus minor* from dogs to human can be possible. Thus, the canine oral microbiome can be zoonotic and oral-to-oral transfer from dogs to human is a possible cause of oral diseases and a risk for the public health. Periodontal diseases have a high prevalence in dogs [66], and it has been demonstrated that *Pasteurella multocida* and *Tannerella forsythia* can be transmitted from animal to human [67–69].

4. Reverse zoonotic disease transmission

Zoonotic diseases have been related with the infection transmission from animals to humans, but some pathogens can be transmitted from humans to animals. Zooanthroponosis, bidirectional zoonosis, anthroponosis, anthropozoonosis, human-to-animal disease transmission and reverse zoonosis are the terms to refer when any human pathogen infects animals. The first transmission of human parasites to animals was published in 2000 [70]. In general, anthropozoonosis and its ecology are poorly studied; however, they are defined as an important health trouble in the world. *Mycobacterium tuberculosis, M. bovis, Staphylococcus aureus,* Methicillin-resistant bacteria, *Streptococcus pneumoniae, Campylobacter* sp., *Salmonella* sp., *Shigella sonnei, S. boydii, S. flexneri, Escherichia coli,* Oxacillin-resistant bacteria and *Helicobacter pylori* are some bacteria that have caused reverse zoonosis in livestock, wildlife and companion animals.

Viruses also have been reported as reverse zoonosis agents, for example, hepatitis E, measles, human metapneumovirus, influenza A (H1N1), rotavirus, human herpesvirus 1 and 4, and human adenovirus A-F have been transmitted from humans to animals. Parasites as *Chilonastix mesnili, Endolimax nana, Strongyloides fuelleborni, Trichuris trichiura, Encephalitozoon intestinalis, Giardia duodenalis, C. parvum, Blastocystis* sp., *Ascaris lumbricoides, T. trichiura* and *Isospora* sp., and fungi as *Microsporum* sp., *Trichophyton* sp., *Tricophyton rubrum, Candida albicans* and *Microsporum gypseum* have been also reported in animal pathogenesis obtained from ill humans [70].

Bacteria (38%) are the prevalent agents of reverse zoonosis and other as viruses (29%), parasites (21%) and fungi (13%) are also involved in human-to-animal disease transmission. This type of transmission has been studied and conducted in all the continents except Antarctica, North America being the region with highest prevalence (**Figure 5**) [70]. The main transmission ways include fomite, oral contact, aerosols and inoculation.

Two patterns of transmission have been defined to describe the transmission from wildlife to humans [71]. In the first one a viral disease from wildlife is rarely transmitted to humans

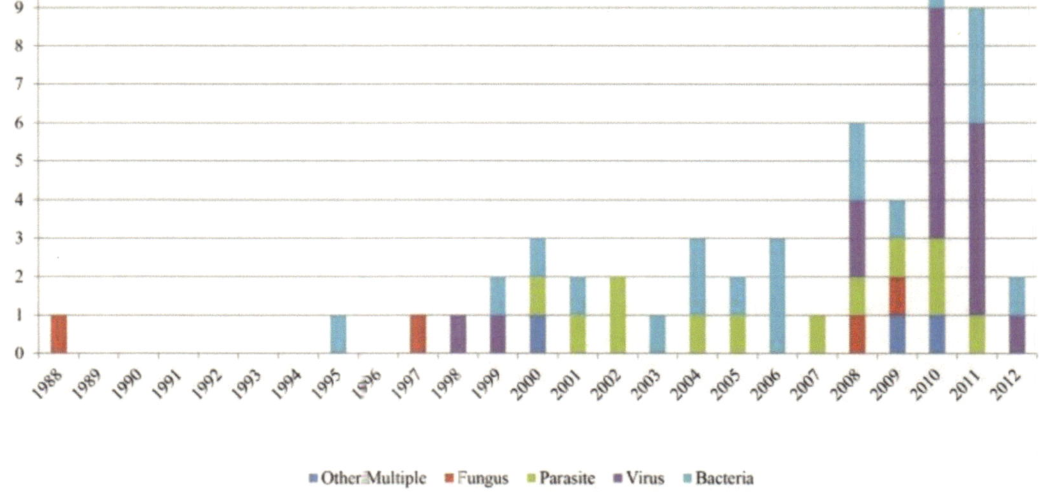

Figure 5. Timeline and frequency of reverse zoonoses publications included in this review shown by pathogen type.

and then that can be horizontally transmitted from humans-to-humans. In this pattern, the virus maintains its cycle in humans. Simian Immunodeficiency virus is the major example of this pattern [72]. The second pattern involves two or more animals and humans, with any arthropod as mediator. In this case, the transmission humans-to-humans is very rare (e.g., West Nile virus) [73].

With the previous background, the diagnosis of reverse zoonosis via metagenomics would bring novel information about the transmission routes, ecology of these zoonosis and anthropozoonosis and serotypes that cause infections in animals. Pathogen bacteria, parasites, viruses and fungi, including those available to produce reverse zoonosis, can be identified by metagenomic profile analysis of ill animals and humans. Metagenomics also can provide novel and useful information about the dynamic and ecology of pathogen populations. Other global studies as transcriptomics can suggest the differential transcriptional levels of pathogens in different hosts. This research will bring important information to design specific therapies for different hosts.

Viruses approximately comprise 200 human pathogen species, and novel pathogen viruses are discovered each year in the rate of two per year [74]. The viral tropism is extensively discussing because some viruses can rapidly jump between species such as avian [75] and swine [76] influenza epidemics. These points are attractive to study viral reverse zoonosis and identify mutations and viral new properties involved in anthropozoonosis. Some authors report that between 36 and 562 viral pathogens remain to be discovered [74]. Probably some of them can cause animal illness.

5. Metagenomic and surveillance programs

As mentioned in the chapter, metagenomics provides a powerful approach to study viromes and microbiomes from different wild, domestic animals and humans. Detection of new and reemerging infectious agents in such hosts not only is a source of information relevant to public health, regarding the ecology and epidemiology of infectious disease, but also allows the establishment of appropriate surveillance programs; mainly in developing countries, to prevent transmission of infectious diseases in humans still remains a threat worldwide.

The increasing of the population represents a large risk to facilite the zoonotic diseases. Also, the distribution of human settlements to regions previously inhabited influence the incidence, geographical distribution and the incorporation of infectious agents, favoring the transmission of infectious diseases. Haagmans and coworkers showed the role of camels in the transmission of Middle East Respiratory Syndrome Coronavirus (MERS-CoV)-to-humans [77]. These dates show the importance on metagenomics studies in animal species that have not been considered as a reservoir of zoonotic agents. In addition, it could improve surveillance programs in infectious diseases, which may include new host such as arthropods, wild and domestic animals.

Epidemiological surveillance programs must be accompanied by economic capacity, infrastructure, research and interdisciplinarity allowing adequate and timely response, to address emerging and reemerging infectious diseases in all countries, especially in developing countries where the incidence of these diseases is increasing. Recent study by Pan American Health Organization (PAHO 2016), which involved the participation of ministries of health in different countries of Latin America, showed that the greatest need in these countries regarding emerging infectious diseases lies in the diagnosis and laboratory capabilities for specific diseases such as rabies, leptospirosis, brucellosis, West Nile virus (WNV), Bovine Spongiform Encephalopathy (BSE), and conditions for surveillance of Ebola virus disease (EVD) and avian influenza (AI) [78].

In this context, metagenomics would be a potential tool for the detection of new species that could potentially be a threat for human health; furthermore, it is used for surveillance of emerging diseases.

6. Conclusions

As analyzed, metagenomics provides a powerful and useful approach to study viromes and microbiomes in animals and humans. The relevant information derived from metagenomic studies provides new highlights about zoonotic diseases and its relationships with human. Due to, metagenomic should be extensive to diagnostic activities in order to identify the presence of new viruses and other zoonotic agents, even human pathogens. Metagenomics also provides information about the structural composition of the microbial populations and communities, and how can change them during different zoonosis. Thus, culture-independent methods open new opportunities in the zoonotic diagnostics because these allow to work with complex samples and describe in detail the associated microbiota and virome.

Author details

Laura Inés Cuervo-Soto[1], Silvio Alejandro López-Pazos[1] and Ramón Alberto Batista-García[2]*

*Address all correspondence to rabg@uaem.mx

1 Departamento de Biología, Facultad de Ciencias, Universidad Antonio Nariño, Bogotá, Colombia

2 Centro de Investigación en Dinámica Celular, Instituto de Investigación en Ciencias Básicas y Aplicadas, Universidad Autónoma del Estado de Morelos, Morelos, Mexico

References

[1] Karesh WB, Dobson A, Lloyd-Smith JO, Lubroth J, Dixon MA, Bennett M, et al. Ecology of zoonoses: Natural and unnatural histories. Lancet. 2012;**380**:1936-1945. DOI: 10.1016/S0140-6736(12)61678-X

[2] Smits SL, Bodewes R, Ruiz-González A, Baumgärtner W, Koopmans MP, Osterhaus AD, Schürch AC. Recovering full-length viral genomes from metagenomes. Frontiers in Microbiology. 2015;**6**:1069. DOI: 10.3389/fmicb.2015.01069

[3] Wang LF, Crameri G. Emerging zoonotic viral diseases. Revue Scientifique et Technique. 2014;**33**(2):569-581 PubMed PMID: 25707184

[4] Cutler SJ, Fooks AR, van der Poel WH. Public health threat of new, reemerging, and neglected zoonoses in the industrialized world. Emerging Infectious Diseases. 2010;**16**(1):1-7. DOI: 10.3201/eid1601.081467

[5] Taylor LH, Latham SM, Woolhouse ME. Risk factors for human disease emergence. Philosophical Transactions of the Royal Society B: Biological Sciences. 2001;**356**(1411):983-989. DOI: 10.1098/rstb.2001.0888

[6] Farahmand M, Nahrevanian H. Application of recombinant proteins for Serodiagnosis of visceral Leishmaniasis in humans and dog. Iranian Biomedical Journal. 2016;**20**(3):128-134. DOI: 10.7508/ibj.2016.03.001

[7] Sun X, Lu H, Jia B, Chang Z, Peng S, Yin J, Chen Q, Jiang N. A comparative study of *Toxoplasma gondii* seroprevalence in three healthy Chinese populations detected using native and recombinant antigens. Parasites & Vectors. 2013;**6**(1):241. DOI: 10.1186/1756-3305-6-241

[8] Razzauti M, Galan M, Bernard M, Maman S, Klopp C, Charbonnel N, Vayssier-Taussat M, Eloit M, Cosson JF. A comparison between Transcriptome sequencing and 16S Metagenomics for detection of bacterial pathogens in wildlife. PLoS Neglected Tropical Diseases. 2015;**9**(8):e0003929. DOI: 10.1371/journal.pntd.0003929

[9] Bexfield N, Kellam P. Metagenomics and the molecular identification of novel viruses. Veterinary Journal. 2011;**190**(2):191-198. DOI: 10.1016/j.tvjl.2010.10.014

[10] Barzon L, Lavezzo E, Militello V, Toppo S, Palù G. Applications of next-generation sequencing technologies to diagnostic virology. International Journal of Molecular Sciences. 2011;**12**(11):7861-7884. DOI: 10.3390/ijms12117861

[11] Mokili JL, Rohwer F, Dutilh BE. Metagenomics and future perspectives in virus discovery. Current Opinion in Virology. 2012;**2**(1):63-77. DOI: 10.1016/j.coviro.2011.12.004

[12] Desai N, Antonopoulos D, Gilbert JA, Glass EM, Meyer F. From genomics to metagenomics. Current Opinion in Biotechnology. 2012;**23**(1):72-76. DOI: 10.1016/j.copbio.2011.12.017

[13] Sturgeon A, Stull JW, Costa MC, Weese JS. Metagenomic analysis of the canine oral cavity as revealed by high-through put pyrosequencing of the 16S rRNA gene. Veterinary Microbiology. 2013;**162**(2-4):891-898. DOI: 10.1016/j.vetmic.2012.11.018

[14] Tun HM, Brar MS, Khin N, Jun L, Hui RK, Dowd SE, Leung FC. Gene-centric metagenomics analysis of feline intestinal microbiome using 454 junior pyrosequencing. Journal of Microbiological Methods. 2012;**88**(3):369-376. DOI: 10.1016/j.mimet.2012.01.001

[15] Blomström AL. Viral metagenomics as an emerging and powerful tool in veterinary medicine. The Veterinary Quarterly. 2011;**31**(3):107-114. DOI: 10.1080/01652176.2011.604971

[16] Kohl C, Brinkmann A, Dabrowski PW, Radonić A, Nitsche A, Kurth A. Protocol for metagenomic virus detection in clinical specimens. Emerging Infectious Diseases. 2015;**21**(1):48-57. DOI: 10.3201/eid2101.140766

[17] Mihalov-Kovács E, Fehér E, Martella V, Bányai K, Farkas SL. The fecal virome of domesticated animals. Virus Disease. 2014;**25**(2):150-157. DOI: 10.1007/s13337-014-0192-1

[18] Temmam S, Davoust B, Berenger JM, Raoult D, Desnues C. Viral metagenomics on animals as a tool for the detection of zoonoses prior to human infection? International Journal of Molecular Sciences. 2014;**15**(6):10377-10397. DOI: 10.3390/ijms150610377

[19] Ng TF, Willner DL, Lim YW, Schmieder R, Chau B, Nilsson C, Anthony S, Ruan Y, Rohwer F, Breitbart M. Broad surveys of DNA viral diversity obtained through viral metagenomics of mosquitoes. PLoS One. 2011;**6**(6):e20579. DOI: 10.1371/journal.pone.0020579

[20] Coffey LL, Page BL, Greninger AL, Herring BL, Russell RC, Doggett SL, Haniotis J, Wang C, Deng X, Delwart EL. Enhanced arbovirus surveillance with deep sequencing: Identification of novel rhabdoviruses and bunyaviruses in Australian mosquitoes. Virology. 2014;**448**:146-158. DOI: 10.1016/j.virol.2013.09.026

[21] Hall-Mendelin S, Allcock R, Kresoje N, van den Hurk AF, Warrilow D. Detection of arboviruses and other micro-organisms in experimentally infected mosquitoes using massively parallel sequencing. PLoS One. 2013;**8**(2):e58026. DOI: 10.1371/journal.pone.0058026

[22] Cook S, Chung BY, Bass D, Moureau G, Tang S, McAlister E, Culverwell CL, Glücksman E, Wang H, Brown TD, Gould EA, Harbach RE, de Lamballerie X, Firth AE. Novel virus discovery and genome reconstruction from field RNA samples reveals highly divergent viruses in dipteran hosts. PLoS One. 2013;**8**(11):e80720. DOI: 10.1371/journal.pone.0080720

[23] Liu S, Vijayendran D, Bonning BC. Next generation sequencing technologies for insect virus discovery. Virus. 2011;**3**(10):1849-1869. DOI: 10.3390/v3101849

[24] Junglen S, Drosten C. Virus discovery and recent insights into virus diversity in arthropods. Current Opinion in Microbiology. 2013;**16**(4):507-513. DOI: 10.1016/j.mib.2013.06.005

[25] Charrel RN, de Lamballerie X. Zoonotic aspects of arenavirus infections. Veterinary Microbiology. 2010;**140**(3-4):213-220. DOI: 10.1016/j.vetmic.2009.08.027

[26] Dacheux L, Cervantes-Gonzalez M, Guigon G, Thiberge JM, Vandenbogaert M, Maufrais C, Caro V, Bourhy H. A preliminary study of viral metagenomics of French bat species in contact with humans: Identification of new mammalian viruses. PLoS One. 2014;**9**(1):e87194. DOI: 10.1371/journal.pone.0087194

[27] Breitbart M, Salamon P, Andresen B, Mahaffy JM, Segall AM, Mead D, Azam F, Rohwer F. Genomic analysis of uncultured marine viral communities. Proceedings of the National Academy of Sciences of the United States of America. 2002;**99**(22):14250-14255. DOI: 10.1073/pnas.202488399

[28] Culley AI, Lang AS, Suttle CA. Metagenomic analysis of coastal RNA virus communities. Science. 2006;**312**(5781):1795-1798. DOI: 10.1126/science.1127404

[29] Breitbart M, Rohwer F. Method for discovering novel DNA viruses in blood using viral particle selection and shotgun sequencing. BioTechniques. 2005;**39**(5):729-736. DOI: 10.2144/000112019

[30] Fancello L, Raoult D, Desnues C. Computational tools for viral metagenomics and their application in clinical research. Virology. 2012;**434**(2):162-174. DOI: 10.1016/j.virol.2012.09.025

[31] Haynes M, Rohwer F. The human virome. In: Nelson KE, editor. Metagenomics of the Human Body. New York, NY: Springer; 2011. pp. 63-77

[32] Pride DT, Salzman J, Haynes M, Rohwer F, Davis-Long C, White RA 3rd, Loomer P, Armitage GC, Relman DA. Evidence of a robust resident bacteriophage population revealed through analysis of the human salivary virome. The ISME Journal. 2012;**6**(5):915-926. DOI: 10.1038/ismej.2011.169

[33] Willner D, Furlan M, Haynes M, Schmieder R, Angly FE, Silva J, Tammadoni S, Nosrat B, Conrad D, Rohwer F. Metagenomic analysis of respiratory tract DNA viral communities in cystic fibrosis and non-cystic fibrosis individuals. PLoS One. 2009;**4**(10):e7370. DOI: 10.1371/journal.pone.0007370

[34] Reyes A, Haynes M, Hanson N, Angly FE, Heath AC, Rohwer F, Gordon JI. Viruses in the faecal microbiota of monozygotic twins and their mothers. Nature. 2010;**466**(7304):334-338. DOI: 10.1038/nature09199

[35] Willner D, Furlan M, Schmieder R, Grasis JA, Pride DT, Relman DA, Angly FE,McDole T, Mariella RP Jr, Rohwer F, Haynes M. Metagenomic detection of phage-encoded platelet-binding factors in the human oral cavity. Proceedings of the National Academy of Sciences of the United States of America. 2011;**108**(Suppl 1):4547-4553. DOI: 10.1073/pnas.1000089107

[36] Weinbauer MG. Ecology of prokaryotic viruses. FEMS Microbiology Reviews. 2004;**28**(2):127-181. DOI: 10.1016/j.femsre.2003.08.001

[37] Breitbart M, Felts B, Kelley S, Mahaffy JM, Nulton J, Salamon P, Rohwer F. Diversity and population structure of a near-shore marine-sediment viral community. Proceedings of the Biological Sciences. 2004;**271**(1539):565-574. DOI: 10.1098/rspb.2003.2628

[38] Fancello L, Desnues C, Raoult D, Rolain JM. Bacteriophages and diffusion of genes encoding antimicrobial resistance in cystic fibrosis sputum microbiota. The Journal of Antimicrobial Chemotherapy. 2011;**66**(11):2448-2454. DOI: 10.1093/jac/dkr315

[39] McMullan LK, Frace M, Sammons SA, Shoemaker T, Balinandi S, Wamala JF, Lutwama JJ, Downing RG, Stroeher U, MacNeil A, Nichol ST. Using next generation sequencing to identify yellow fever virus in Uganda. Virology. 2012;**422**(1):1-5. DOI: 10.1016/j.virol.2011.08.024

[40] Greninger AL, Chen EC, Sittler T, Scheinerman A, Roubinian N, Yu G, Kim E, Pillai DR, Guyard C, Mazzulli T, Isa P, Arias CF, Hackett J, Schochetman G, Miller S, Tang P, Chiu CY.

A metagenomic analysis of pandemic influenza A (2009 H1N1) infection in patients from North America. PLoS One. 2010;**5**(10):e13381. DOI: 10.1371/journal.pone.0013381

[41] Thurber RV, Haynes M, Breitbart M, Wegley L, Rohwer F. Laboratory procedures to generate viral metagenomes. Nature Protocols. 2009;**4**(4):470-483. DOI: 10.1038/nprot.2009.10

[42] Kim KH, Bae JW. Amplification methods bias metagenomic libraries of uncultured single-stranded and double-stranded DNA viruses. Applied and Environmental Microbiology. 2011;**77**(21):7663-7668. DOI: 10.1128/AEM.00289-11

[43] Kim MS, Park EJ, Roh SW, Bae JW. Diversity and abundance of single-stranded DNA viruses in human feces. Applied and Environmental Microbiology. 2011;**77**(22):8062-8070. DOI: 10.1128/AEM.06331-11

[44] Ghosh TS, Mohammed MH, Komanduri D, Mande SS. ProViDE: A software tool for accurate estimation of viral diversity in metagenomic samples. Bioinformation. 2011;**6**(2):91-94

[45] Roux S, Faubladier M, Mahul A, Paulhe N, Bernard A, Debroas D, Enault F. Metavir: A web server dedicated to virome analysis. Bioinformatics. 2011;**27**(21):3074-3075. DOI: 10.1093/bioinformatics/btr519

[46] Lorenzi HA, Hoover J, Inman J, Safford T, Murphy S, Kagan L, Williamson SJ. TheViral MetaGenome annotation pipeline (VMGAP):An automated tool for the functional annotation of viral metagenomic shotgun sequencing data. Standards in Genomic Sciences. 2011;**4**(3):418-429. DOI: 10.4056/sigs.1694706

[47] Stang A, Korn K, Wildner O, Uberla K. Characterization of virus isolates by particle-associated nucleic acid PCR. Journal of Clinical Microbiology. 2005;**43**(2):716-720

[48] Capobianchi MR, Giombini E, Rozera G. Next-generation sequencing technology in clinical virology. Clinical Microbiology and Infection. 2013;**19**(1):15-22. DOI: 10.1111/1469-0691.12056

[49] Belák S, Karlsson OE, Blomström AL, Berg M, Granberg F. New viruses in veterinary medicine, detected by metagenomic approaches. Veterinary Microbiology. 2013;**165**(1-2): 95-101. DOI: 10.1016/j.vetmic.2013.01.022

[50] Dinsdale EA, Edwards RA, Hall D, Angly F, Breitbart M, et al. Functional metagenomic profiling of nine biomes. Nature. 2008;**452**(7187):629-632. DOI: 10.1038/nature06810

[51] Handelsman J. Metagenomics: Application of genomics to uncultured microorganisms. Microbiology and Molecular Biology Reviews. 2004;**68**(4):669-685. DOI: 10.1128/MMBR.68.4.669-685.2004

[52] Qu A, Brulc JM, Wilson MK, Law BF, Theoret JR, et al. Comparative metagenomics reveals host specific metavirulomes and horizontal gene transfer elements in the chicken cecum microbiome. PLoS One. 2008;**3**(8):e2945. DOI: 10.1371/journal.pone.0002945

[53] Hatta Y, Omatsu T, Tsuchiaka S, Katayama Y, Taniguchi S, Masangkay JS, Puentespina R Jr, Eres E, Une Y, Yoshikawa Y, Maeda K, Kyuwa S, Mizutani T. Detection of *Campylobacter*

jejuni in rectal swab samples from *Rousettus amplexicaudatus* in the Philippines. The Journal of Veterinary Medical Science. 2016;**78**(8):1347-1350. DOI: 10.1292/jvms.15-0621

[54] Schipper J, Chanson JS, Chiozza F, Cox NA, Hoffmann M, Katariya V, Lamoreux J, Rodrigues AS, Stuart SN. The status of the world's land and marine mammals: Diversity, threat, and knowledge. Science. 2008;**322**(5899):225-230. DOI: 10.1126/science.1165115

[55] Gibbons RV. Cryptogenic rabies, bats, and the question of aerosol transmission. Annals of Emergency Medicine. 2002;**39**(5):528-536

[56] Chua KB, Koh CL, Hooi PS, Wee KF, Khong JH, Chua BH, Chan YP, Lim ME, Lam SK. Isolation of Nipah virus from Malaysian Island flying-foxes. Microbes and Infection. 2002;**4**(2):145-151

[57] Chua KB, Bellini WJ, Rota PA, Harcourt BH, Tamin A, Lam SK, Ksiazek TG, Rollin PE, Zaki SR, Shieh W, Goldsmith CS, Gubler DJ, Roehrig JT, Eaton B, Gould AR, Olson J, Field H, Daniels P, Ling AE, Peters CJ, Anderson LJ, Mahy BW. Nipah virus: A recently emergent deadly paramyxovirus. Science. 2000;**288**(5470):1432-1435. DOI: 10.1126/science.288.5470.1432

[58] Murray K, Rogers R, Selvey L, Selleck P, Hyatt A, Gould A, Gleeson L, Hooper P, Westbury H. A novel morbillivirus pneumonia of horses and its transmission to humans. Emerging Infectious Diseases. 1995;**1**(1):31-33. DOI: 10.3201/eid0101.950107

[59] Badrane H, Bahloul C, Perrin P, Tordo N. Evidence of two Lyssavirus phylogroups with distinct pathogenicity and immunogenicity. Journal of Virology. 2001;**75**(7):3268-3276. DOI: 10.1128/JVI.75.7.3268-3276.2001

[60] Reyes AW, Rovira HG, Masangkay JS, Ramirez TJ, Yoshikawa Y. Baticados WN, Polymerase chain reaction assay and conventional isolation of Salmonella spp. from Philippine bats. Acta Scientiae Veterinariae. 2011;**39**:947

[61] Klite PD. Intestinal bacterial flora and transit time of three neotropical bat species. Journal of Bacteriology. 1965;**90**:375-9

[62] Kay GL, Sergeant MJ, Giuffra V, Bandiera P, Milanese M, Bramanti B, Bianucci R, Pallen MJ. Recovery of a medieval *Brucella melitensis* genome using shotgun Metagenomics. MBio. 2014;**5**(4):e01337-14). DOI: 10.1128/mBio.01337-14

[63] Marsh PD. Microbial ecology of dental plaque and its significance in health and disease. Advances in Dental Research. 1994;**8**:263-271. DOI: 10.1177/08959374940080022001

[64] Fowler EB, Breault LG, Cuenin MF. Periodontal disease and its association with systemic disease. Military Medicine. 2001;**166**:85-89

[65] Oh C, Lee K, Cheong Y, Lee SW, Park SY, Song CS, Choi IS, Lee JB. Comparison of the oral microbiomes of canines and their owners using next-generation sequencing. PLoS One. 2015;**10**(7):e0131468. DOI: 10.1371/journal.pone.0131468

[66] Harvey CE, Thornsberry C, Miller BR. Subgingival bacteria—Comparison of culture results in dogs and cats with gingivitis. Journal of Veterinary Dentistry. 1995;**12**:147-150

[67] Booij-Vrieling HE, van der Reijden WA, Houwers DJ, de Wit WE, Bosch-Tijhof CJ, Penning LC, van Winkelhoff AJ, Hazewinkel HA. Comparison of periodontal pathogens between cats and their owners. Veterinary Microbiology. 2010;**144**(1-2):147-152. DOI: 10.1016/j.vetmic.2009.12.046

[68] Oehler RL, Velez AP, Mizrachi M, Lamarche J, Gompf S. Bite-related and septic syndromes caused by cats and dogs. The Lancet Infectious Diseases. 2009;**9**(7):439-447. DOI: 10.1016/S1473-3099(09)70110-0

[69] Yamasaki Y, Nomura R, Nakano K, Naka S, Matsumoto-Nakano M, Asai F, et al. Distribution of period ontopathic bacterial species in dogs and their owners. Archives of Oral Biology. 2012;**57**(9):1183-1188. DOI: 10. 1016/j.archoralbio.2012.02.015

[70] Messenger AM, Barnes AN, Gray GC. Reverse zoonotic disease transmission (zooanthroponosis): A systematic review of seldom-documented human biological threats to animals. PLoS One. 2014;**9**(2):e89055. DOI: 10.1371/journal.pone.0089055

[71] Bengis RG, Leighton FA, Fischer JR, Artois M, Mörner T, Tate CM. The role of wildlife in emerging and re-emerging zoonoses. Revue Scientifique et Technique. 2004;**23**(2):497-511

[72] Hahn BH, Shaw GM, De Cock KM, Sharp PM. AIDS as a zoonosis: Scientific and public health implications. Science. 2000;**287**(5453):607-614

[73] Trevejo RT, Eidson M. Zoonosis update West Nile virus. Journal of the American Veterinary Medical Association. 2008;**232**(9):1302-1309. DOI: 10.2460/javma.232.9.1302

[74] Woolhouse ME, Howey R, Gaunt E, Reilly L, Chase-Topping M, Savill N. Temporal trends in the discovery of human viruses. Proceedings of the Biological Sciences. 2008;**275**(1647):2111-2115. DOI: 10.1098/rspb.2008.0294

[75] Ungchusak K, Auewarakul P, Dowell SF, Kitphati R, Auwanit W, Puthavathana P, Uiprasertkul M, Boonnak K, Pittayawonganon C, Cox NJ, Zaki SR, Thawatsupha P, Chittaganpitch M, Khontong R, Simmerman JM, Chunsutthiwat S. Probable person-to-person transmission of avian influenza a (H5N1). The New England Journal of Medicine. 2005;**352**(4):333-340

[76] Smith GJ, Vijaykrishna D, Bahl J, Lycett SJ, Worobey M, Pybus OG, Ma SK, Cheung CL, Raghwani J, Bhatt S, Peiris JS, Guan Y, Rambaut A. Origins and evolutionary genomics of the 2009 swine-origin H1N1 influenza A epidemic. Nature. 2009;**459**(7250):1122-1125. DOI: 10.1038/nature08182

[77] Haagmans BL, Al Dhahiry SH, Reusken CB, Raj VS, Galiano M, Myers R, et al. Middle East respiratory syndrome coronavirus in dromedary camels: An outbreak investigation. The Lancet Infectious Diseases. 2014;**14**(2):140-145. DOI: 10.1016/S1473-3099(13)70690-X

[78] Preliminary report1. A survey of zoonoses programmes in the americas. PAHO. 2016. http://www.paho.org/panaftosa/index.php?option=com_docman&task=doc_download&gid=488&itemid=311